The Hoofcare Companion

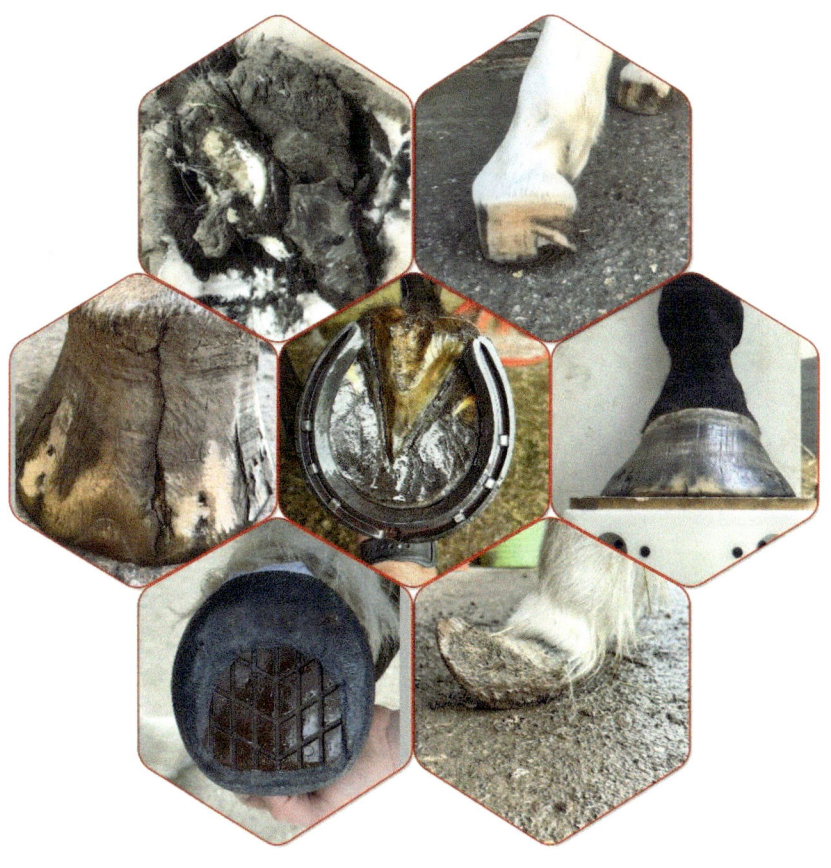

Marc Jerram

Copyright

© 2023 by Marc Jerram All rights reserved.

No part of this publication may be reproduced, distributed or transmitted in any form or by any means, including photocopying, recording, or other electronic or mechanical methods, without the prior written permission of the author, except in the case of brief quotations embodied in critical reviews and certain other non-commercial uses permitted by copyright law. Neither the author nor the publisher assumes any responsibility or liability whatsoever on behalf of the consumer or reader of this material. The resources in this book are provided for informational purposes only and should not be used to replace the specialized training and professional judgment of their own farrier or veterinarian. Neither the author nor the publisher can be held responsible for the use of the information provided within this book. Please, always consult a trained professional before making any decision regarding treatment of your horse or others.

La Tour, Old Weston Road, Bishops Wood, Staffordshire, ST19 9AG, United Kingdom.

marcsforge@hotmail.com

ISBN 978-1-3999-6097-7

Acknowledgements

There are many farriers and vets I have worked with over the years, and I would like to say thank you to you all for sharing your knowledge so freely and allowing me to develop my skills and experience. There are many horses documented in this book and it is of great gratitude to the owners of these horses for allowing me to work on and document their horses so that other horses can be helped in the future. A huge thanks go to my proofreaders Dr Beth Bromley MRCVS and David Hall BSc (Hons) DipWCF (Hons) for checking the content and their advice. Finally, I would like to thank my family for allowing me the time to complete this project over the last year, this book could not have been possible without their support.

CONTENTS

	Pages
Introduction	1 - 3
Chapter 1 – The anatomy of the hoof	4 - 21
Chapter 2 – Care and management of the hoof	22 - 43
Chapter 3 – The role of nutrition in the hoof	44 - 63
Chapter 4 – Conformational faults – birth to maturity	64 - 85
Chapter 5 – Static and dynamic assessment of the hoof	86 - 109
Chapter 6 – Conditions involving hoof imbalance	110 - 121
Chapter 7 – Issues involving equine locomotion	122 - 131
Chapter 8 – Conditions of the soft tissues	132 - 139
Chapter 9 – Conditions of the pedal bone and coffin joint	140 - 161
Chapter 10 – Conditions of the sole	162 - 169
Chapter 11 – Conditions of the frog	170 - 183
Chapter 12 – Conditions of the hoof wall	184 - 201
Chapter 13 – Conditions of the white line	202 - 215
Glossary	216 - 218
Index	219 - 222

Introduction

The inspiration from writing this book came from the lack of reliable information when dealing with a hoof care emergency. Indeed, in the age of internet search engines and social media, anyone and everyone with an opinion have the ability to give advice which has often led to poor outcomes for horses. The case studies detailed in this book provide the reader with firsthand experience and the outcomes that were achieved. The purpose of this book is to help educate new and existing horse owners regarding the common issues that can develop in or around your horse's hoof. It is hoped the information laid out ahead is easy to understand and implement into the daily routine of horse care. During the last 25 years, there have been a marked decrease in the number of riding schools and training centres for new horse owners. This has led to a number of people acquiring horses with the best of intentions but without the pre ownership equine experience and methods that have been passed down through generations. The same can be said for the hoof care of their horses. Whilst every farrier is happy to help educate owners on feet, they can't be there all the time and this is where this book will come in useful, being stored at their stables to act as a first point of reference should a hoof emergency occur.

Although there is a vast amount of information and advice available freely on the internet, much of it is either written by the less experienced or with a marketing strategy towards a certain product. The lameness cases detailed ahead involved a team of people working together for the betterment of the horse. This included the farrier, veterinarian, physiotherapist, saddle fitter and horse owner. There are many situations where the failure to work as a team can lead to a negative outcome for the horse so the author would strongly advise that when looking to select a professional to work on your horse that you select one that is happy to work alongside fellow paraprofessionals, is approachable and is involved in Continual Professional Development (CPD).

The techniques learned to overcome these lameness cases are a result of years of post-graduate study from completing a Bachelor of science degree in Farriery Science at the University of Central Lancashire and a Graduate diploma in Equine locomotor research at the Royal Veterinary College. Not only were many techniques learned in the courses, but the huge network of fellow farriers and paraprofessionals meant that we were able to discuss many cases and help to resolve them successfully. During my career I have been very fortunate to work alongside a number of veterinary practices on the most complicated and challenging of cases. This has then led to the opportunity to teach at a veterinary college and present at many conferences to farriers, vets, physiotherapists and horse owners. The opportunity to stand up in front of large audiences and share my findings to help improve equine welfare is one of the greatest honours you can do.

Detailed in this book are general guidelines on how to maintain hooves free from lameness and pathology. This is what I feel is incredibly important as most textbooks focus on being reactive to a pathology rather than being proactive to prevent it occurring in the first place. These preventative steps include how the horse's diet and nutrition can affect the health of the hoof and the horse. This is a subject that has had little discussion previously and whilst this is a subject that is constantly evolving, the baseline knowledge described later in this book can help to expand your knowledge and establish a good foundational nutrition plan for the health of the hoof.

The use of modern technology to assess horses is something we now have the advantage of using and help to train our own eye. Groundbreaking systems using Inertia Measuring Units (IMU) and Artificial Intelligence (AI) are described as to their use in hoof care and optimising equine performance. The intricate details can help to detect issues early and if used responsibly can be used as a comparative of the horse's movement over time.

The evolution of knowledge of the hoof has advanced over the last 50 years, so many ideas have been disproven or considered not relative to the modern horse although the basic core fundamentals remain the same. Detailed at the end of each chapter is a list of references that have given the author the inspiration to discover the subject further, it is hoped the reader can use this list to further their own knowledge, see a different perspective and formulate their own methods in relation to horses in their care. There are a number of high quality images that have been captured over many years, so many hooves I couldn't put down until I had obtained a photo and demonstrate the progress over a few months.

Whilst this book can be used as a reference point for a particular problem, the reader will find every chapter informative and educational. By the time the book is complete, many new techniques and tips will have been learned to help prevent lameness and improve hoof quality.

Marc Jerram BSc (Hons) Grad Dip ELR CJF AWCF Master Farrier

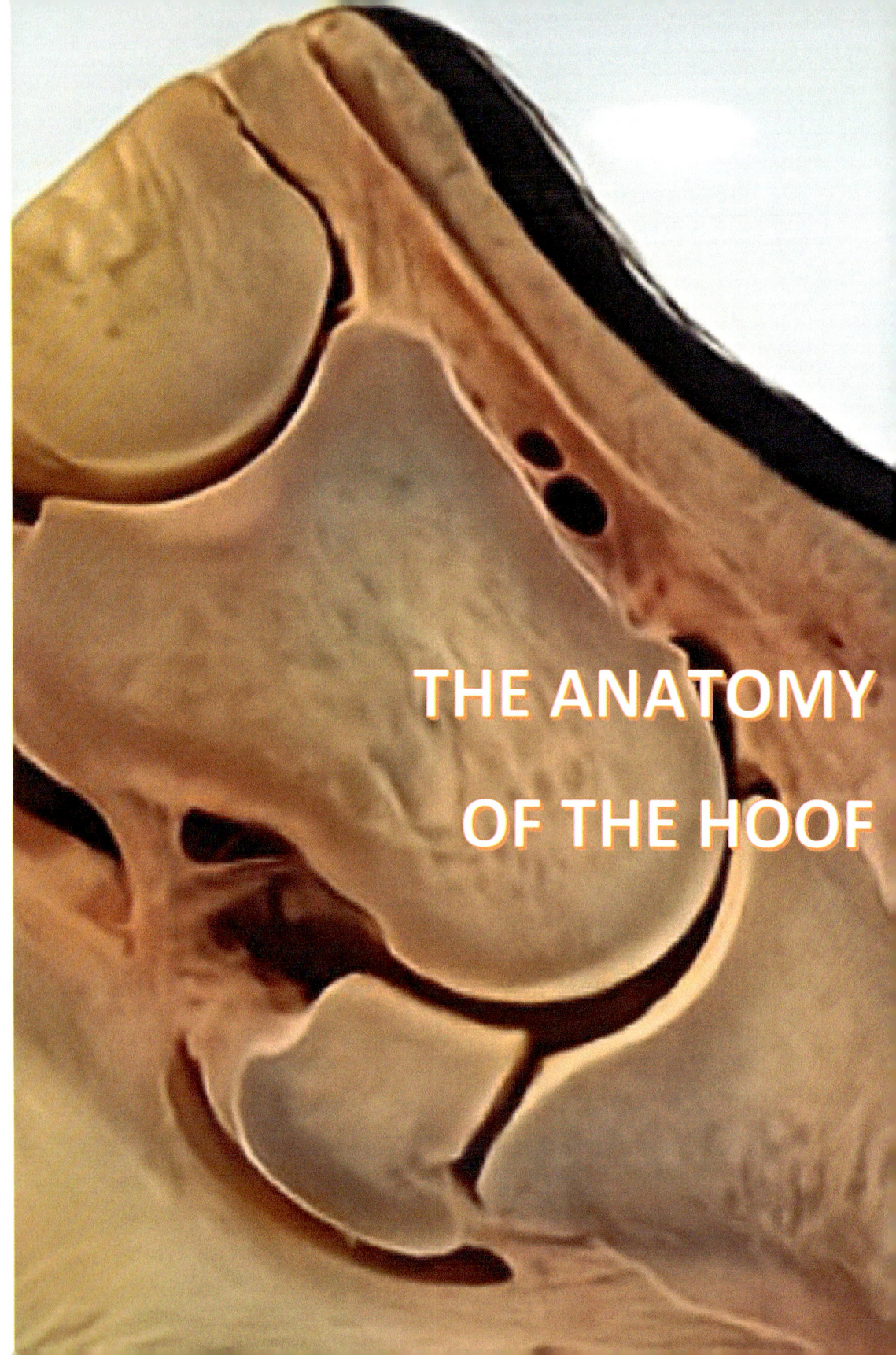

Chapter 1 - The anatomy of the hoof

Introduction

The horse's foot is made up of hoof, elastic, ligament, joint and sensitive structures that are uniquely designed to bear weight, absorb shock, resist wear, regenerate, help to provide traction and assist in pumping venous blood supply. The foot must be kept healthy to operate at peak efficiency.

The hoof is made up of soft and hard horn depending on their primary function. For example, the hoof wall and sole are described as hard horn as they are designed in a way to be tough and resistant to wear while supporting weight. Whereas the frog, white line and periople are soft horn structures that offer flexibility and absorption of concussion as their primary function.

Parts of the hoof

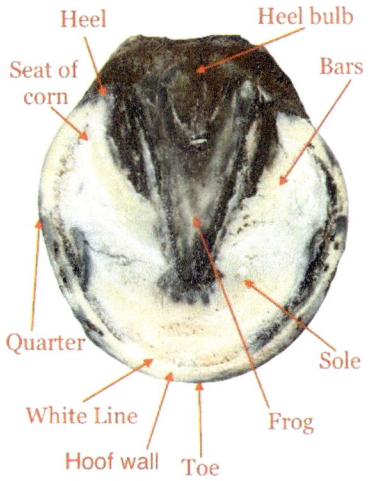

Frog - This is a wedged shaped mass of elastic horn that occupies the area between the bars and sole. The ground surface has a central cleft that opens the sweat glands of the digital cushion. The frog contains around 40% moisture that accounts for its soft pliable state.

White line - The white line is a flexible junction between sole and hoof wall. The white line consists of light coloured horny laminae and has around 28% moisture content.

The anatomy of the hoof

Hoof wall – This is the part of the hoof that can be seen on the ground. It varies in height and thickness from toe to heel with its main function to offer protection to the underlying sensitive structures.

Bars – Bars appear as ridges on the ground surface of the hoof between the sole and frog. These provide stability to the heels and allow for expansion and contraction of the hoof.

Sole – The sole makes up the greater part of the ground bearing surface of the hoof. The sole aids in protecting underlying sensitive structures and dispensing concussion. The moisture content is around 33% and should ideally be a concave or arched shape to function well. The area between the sole and bars is referred to as the seat of corn which can become bruised if the hoof is not functioning well.

Heel bulbs – These are formed by the digital cushion and are covered in skin and periople. Their function is to disperse energy and concussion along with providing flexibility.

Toe – Reference point to the front of the hoof at the midline.

Quarter – Reference point of the widest part of the hoof where most of the flexibility of the hoof originates from during weight bearing.

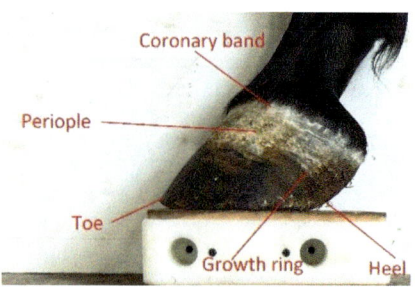

Heel – Reference point to the rear terminal point of the hoof wall.

Periople – Periople is the flexible junction between skin and hoof wall that protects the coronary band from dirt and infection. Periople can also act as a moisture regulator when the hooves have to adapt to a variety of environments. Periople is made up of 40% moisture content and is thickest at the top of the hoof wall before gradually disintegrating as it descends the hoof wall.

Coronary band – The coronary band is a collective name for all the structures which from the upper third of the horny hoof. The coronary band can be described as a highly vascular part of the hoof due to the high amount of blood vessels present.

The coronary band is made up of the coronary corium, coronary cushion and coronary groove that supply nourishment to help grow new hoof wall and laminae.

The anatomy of the hoof

Limb planes of reference

The planes of reference indicate a certain body part, region or direction in any part of the horse. They are used when describing an issue or injury so that a plan can be formulated for recovery or discussion.

Lateral view of the horse

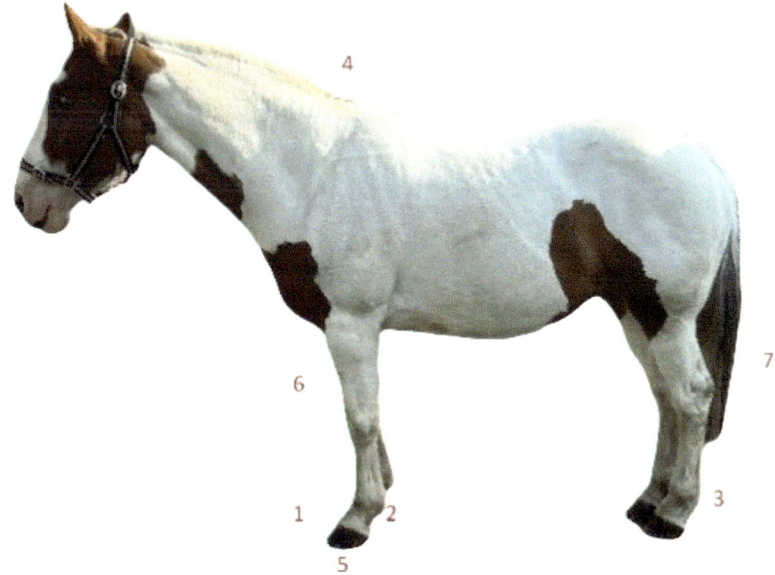

1. Dorsal – Towards the front of the hoof/limb.
2. Palmar – Towards the rear of the front hoof/limb
3. Plantar – Towards the rear of the hind hoof/limb.
4. Proximal – Towards the body in an upward direction from a body segment.
5. Distal – Towards the ground from a body segment.
6. Cranial – Towards the front of the horse, above the knee.
7. Caudal – Towards the rear of the horse, above the knee.

The anatomy of the hoof

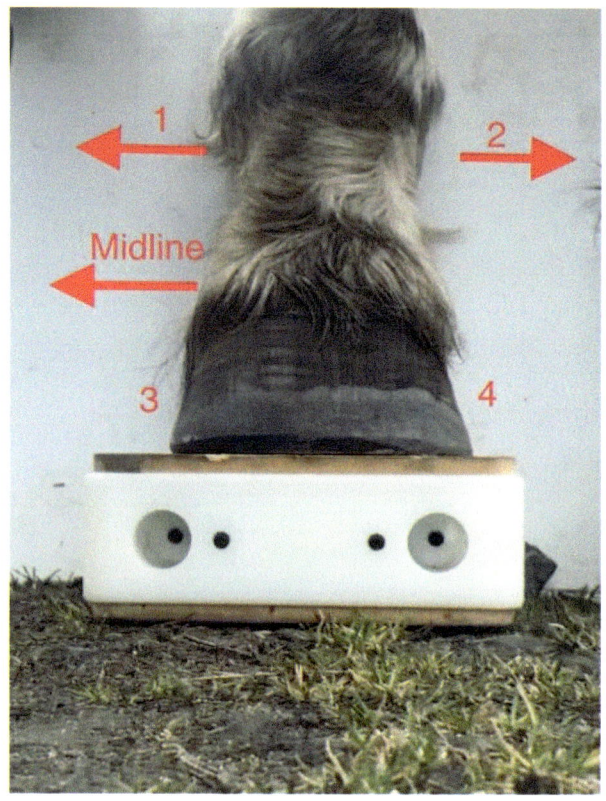

1. Axial - Towards the axis (midline of horse).
2. Abaxial - Away from the axis (midline of horse).
3. Medial - The inside or towards the centre of the horse.
4. Lateral - The outside or furthest away from the centre of the horse.

The anatomy of the hoof

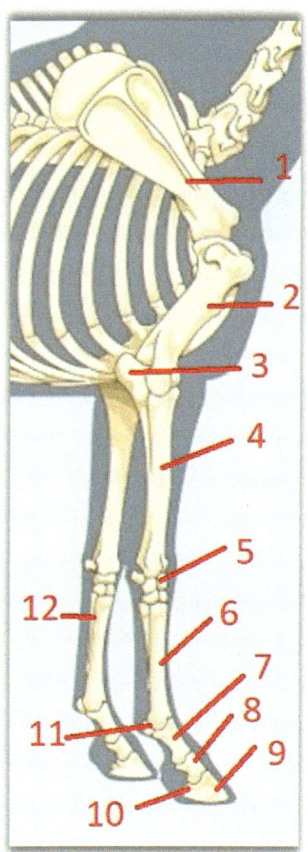

Bones of the forelimb:

1. Scapula
2. Humerus
3. Ulna
4. Radius
5. Carpus (knee)
6. 3rd Metacarpal (cannon bone)
7. Proximal phalanx (long pastern bone)
8. Middle phalanx (short pastern bone)
9. Distal phalanx (coffin bone)
10. Distal sesamoid (navicular bone)
11. Proximal sesamoids (x2)
12. 2nd and 4th metacarpals (splint bones)

The anatomy of the hoof

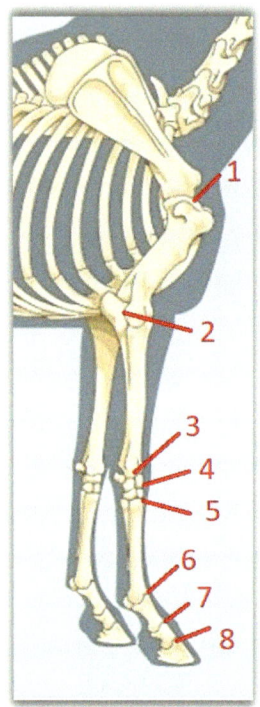

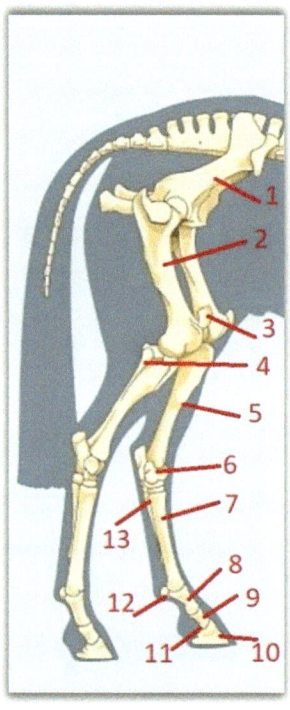

Joints of the forelimb:

1. Shoulder
2. Elbow
3. Radiocarpal
4. Intercarpal
5. Carpometacarpal
6. Metacarpo-phalangeal (fetlock)
7. Proximal interphalangeal (pastern)
8. Distal interphalangeal (coffin)

Bones of the hindlimb:

1. Pelvis (ilium)
2. Femur
3. Patella
4. Fibula
5. Tibia
6. Tarsus (hock)
7. Third metatarsal (cannon)
8. Proximal phalanx (long pastern)
9. Middle phalanx (short pastern)
10. Distal phalanx (coffin)
11. Distal sesamoid (navicular)
12. Proximal sesamoids (x2)
13. 2nd and 4th metatarsals (splint bones)

The anatomy of the hoof

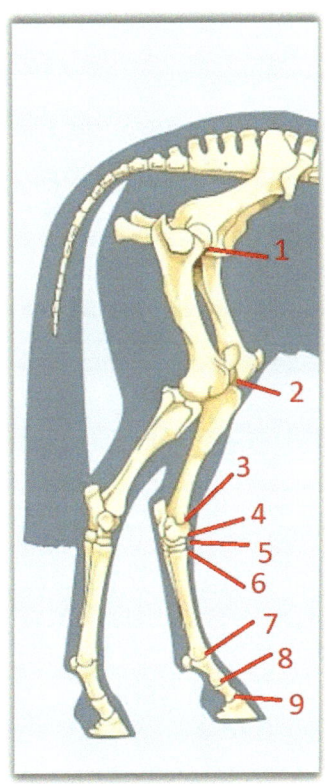

Bones of the foot

There are 3 bones and 1 joint within the hoof. The lower half of the short pastern bone also known as the middle phalanx or P2 is found within the hoof. The coffin bone within the hoof is described as similar to a body within a coffin. Other terms for the coffin bone include pedal bone, distal phalanx or P3. The navicular bone or distal sesamoid is found at the rear of the short pastern and coffin bone with the 3 bones making up the coffin joint.

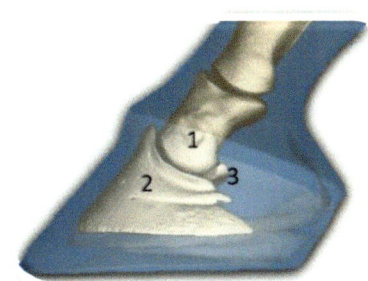

The bones of the foot – 1. Short pastern bone 2. Coffin bone 3. Navicular bone*

Joints of the hindlimb:

1. Hip
2. Stifle
3. Tibio-tarsal
4. Proximal intertarsal
5. Distal intertarsal
6. Tarso-metatarsal
7. Metatarso-phalangeal (fetlock)
8. Proximal interphalangeal (pastern)
9. Distal interphalangeal (coffin)

Tendons of the foot

Muscles and tendons work together to provide movement and assist in providing stability to the limb. A tendon is made up of a tough fibrous band of

The anatomy of the hoof

collagen fibres that act as extensions to the muscles of the body. There are two tendons in the horse's foot, the deep digital flexor tendon found at the rear of the limb passes over the navicular bone and bursa before inserting onto the semi lunar crescent on the base of the coffin bone. The common digital extensor tendon inserts onto the extensor process of the coffin bone.

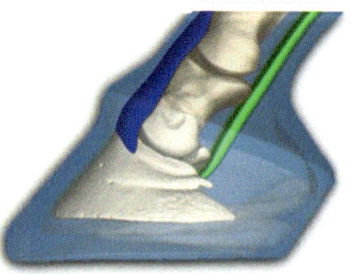

Common digital extensor tendon (blue) and deep digital flexor tendon (green). *

Cartilages of the foot

The horse's foot contains two hyaline cartilages that help absorb ground concussion and allow the rear of the hoof to expand and contract. The hyaline cartilages have a smooth surface with minimal friction, there is no blood supply to this area, so the nutrition is derived from the underlying bone. These cartilages are attached either side of the coffin bone and are often referred to as collateral cartilages.

The collateral cartilages extend dorsally towards the extensor process and palmarly towards the digital cushion. About half of the collateral cartilages extend above the coronary border where they can be palpated, the other half is enclosed within the hoof and extends distally towards the lower half of the coffin bone.

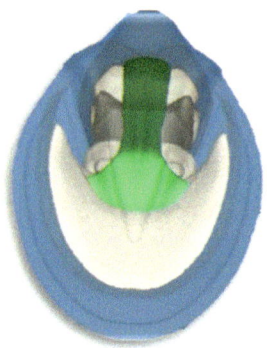

Insertion of the Deep digital flexor tendon onto the semi lunar line of the coffin bone. *

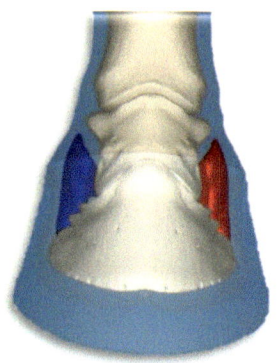

Blue (medial) and red (lateral) cartilages of the hoof. *

The anatomy of the hoof

Cushions of the foot

There are two fibrous fatty cushions found within the hoof that help to absorb concussion and protect the underlying coria. The coronary cushion is found within the coronary band body of sensitive structures and the digital cushion found in the rear of the hoof.

The coronary cushion is covered in papillae and is found on the inner aspect of the coronary groove. This thick, half round fibro-cartilaginous roll forms part of the flexible junction between the hoof and leg and mirrors the shape of the coronary groove.

The digital cushion is made up of 70% moisture and creates a large mass above the frog towards the heels. It contains elastic fibres, as well as collagen and fat cells. The dorsal surface is applied to the deep digital flexor tendon and the palmar surface is moulded onto the corium of the frog. The digital cushion effectively forms a flexible tissue filling the back of the hoof that helps to absorb initial ground impact and help with venous blood return from the hoof.

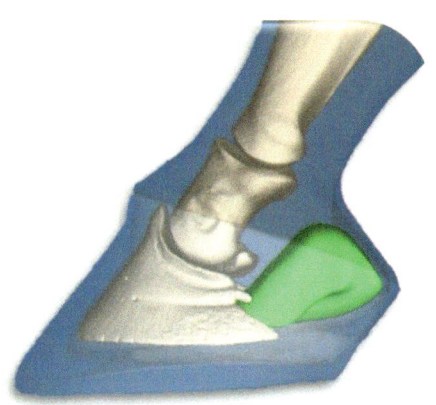

Digital cushion (green) found at the rear of the foot. *

Coria of the foot

There are 5 coria found within the foot that produce and nourish new horn growth. Every part of the hoof grows as a result of cell division in the horn producing cell layer of these coria. The growth of the hoof can be influenced by a variety of factors such as diet or disease.

The perioplic corium develops the periople seen on the hoof wall from small hair like projections (2-3mm in depth) called papillae.

The coronary corium grows the hoof wall from longer papillae (6mm in depth) than those found in the perioplic corium.

13

The anatomy of the hoof

The laminar corium doesn't have papillae but instead bears the primary and secondary sensitive laminae. The sensitive laminae interdigitate with the horny laminae to suspend the horse's bodyweight within the hoof.

The solar corium is attached to the solar surface of the coffin bone and produces horny sole from short papillae (1mm) on which horny sole tubules develop.

The frog corium develops horn from long papillae associated with the digital cushion.

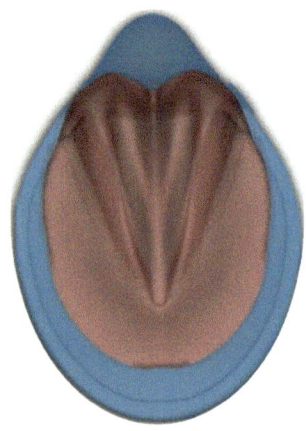

The sole corium found underneath the live sole produces new sole horn. The terminal papillae found on the edges of the sensitive laminae produce new laminae and white line. The frog corium found below the live frog creates new frog horn. *

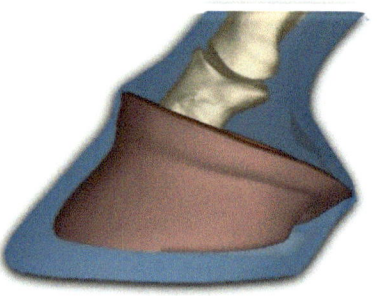

The perioplic corium found at the top of the foot produces new periople. The coronary corium found just underneath the perioplic corium produces the hoof wall. *

Arteries and veins of the foot

The blood supply of the horse carries out a variety of vital functions. The horse has an average of 7-8% of its bodyweight in litres of blood in their arteries and veins. Therefore, a 500KG horse can have between 35 – 40 litres of blood. This is comprised of:

- Plasma – This regulates blood clotting and contains antibodies along with providing nutrition to the cells of the body.

The anatomy of the hoof

- Red blood cells – These contain haemoglobin which provides oxygen to the tissues.
- White blood cells – Primarily associated with fighting infections and produce antibodies.
- Platelets – These have a function of blood clotting.

The horse's foot contains 4 pairs of arteries and veins which make their way into the foot from the pastern. Oxygenated arterial blood travels down into the hoof into the tissues by the capillary network and returns back up the limb becoming deoxygenated venous blood by the way of the veins.

Arteries

The palmar common digital artery is the main supply of blood to the limb and foot. This is referred to as the plantar common digital artery in the hind limbs. This descends medially down the cannon bone and divides into medial and lateral digital arteries just above the fetlock.

The medial and lateral digital arteries are the bilateral supply to the lower limb and hoof that descend down the limb and enter the solear foramina on the coffin bone to help form the terminal arch of arteries. The terminal arch itself connects the digital arteries together within the semi lunar sinus of the coffin bone.

The artery to the digital cushion is the bilateral supply to the structures found at the rear third of the hoof.

The circumflex artery is found on the distal border of the coffin bone where ten communicating branches connect the terminal artery to the circumflex artery. This provides supply to the distal extremity of the foot.

The dorsal distal phalangeal artery travels along the parietal groove of the coffin bone and supplies blood to the laminae.

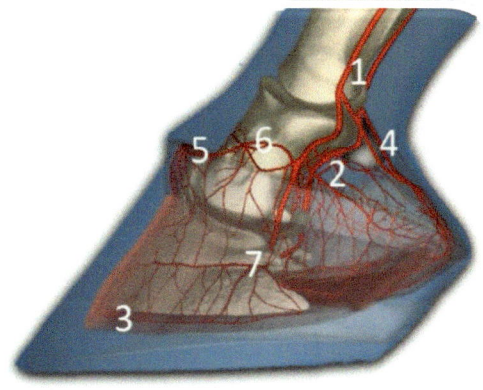

Arteries of the lower limb *

1. Lateral palmar digital artery
2. Medial palmar digital artery
3. Circumflex artery
4. Artery to the digital cushion

The anatomy of the hoof

5. Coronary artery
6. Artery branch to the middle phalanx
7. Dorsal digital phalangeal artery

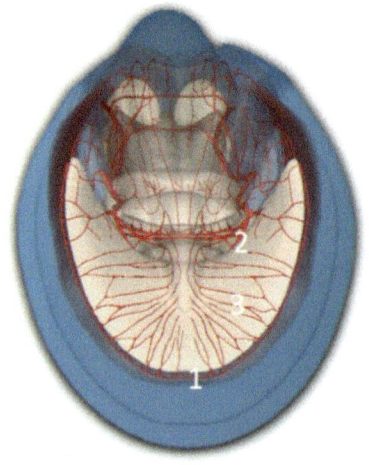

Arteries of the hoof *

1. Circumflex artery
2. Terminal arch
3. Communicating branches

Veins

There are 3 times more veins than arteries within the hoof with most of these being valveless since weight bearing is used for effective venous return from the digit.

The medial and lateral digital veins are the bilateral return from the hoof and lower limb.

The coronary vein returns blood from the coronary band and surrounding structures into the digital veins. Attached to the coronary vein is the coronary venous plexus which is a complex web like structure that serve as important drainage systems for venous blood. The coronary venous plexus is found either side of the collateral cartilages of the coffin bone which assist in bilateral return to the coronary vein and digital veins.

The solar venous plexus is influenced by the movement of the horny sole. The circumflex vein assists in draining the solar surface around the distal border of the coffin bone towards the digital veins.

The frog venous plexus is linked to the caudal vein that helps return blood from the rear third of the foot.

The dorsal vein drains surrounding laminal sensitive laminae and the parietal surface of the coffin bone.

The anatomy of the hoof

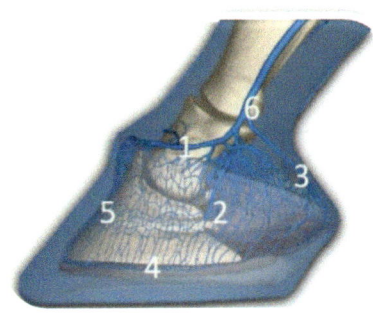

Veins of the lower limb and hoof *

1. Coronary vein with connecting coronary venous plexus
2. Dorsal vein
3. Caudal hoof vein
4. Circumflex vein with connecting solar venous plexus
5. Laminal venous plexus
6. Lateral palmar digital vein

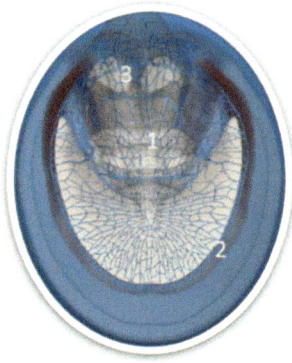

Veins of the foot *

1. Frog venous plexus
2. Circumflex vein with connecting solar venous plexus
3. Caudal hoof vein

Nerves of the foot

The nerve system of the foot is responsible for involuntary reactions when the hoof contacts the ground. The peripheral nerves are white cord like structures that conduct impulses away from and back to the central nervous system. From the spinal cord the larger insulated nerves divide and subdivide as they pass to the extremities of the body.

Peripheral nerves may be efferent or afferent in function. An efferent nerve conducts impulses away from the central nervous system in response to the messages received leading to the muscles contracting and creating movement of the limb. An afferent nerve conducts sensory impulses to the central nervous system in response to different kinds of stimuli received such as touch, heat or pain.

As there are no muscles below the knee and hock, all nerves in the lower limb and hoof are afferent in their function.

The anatomy of the hoof

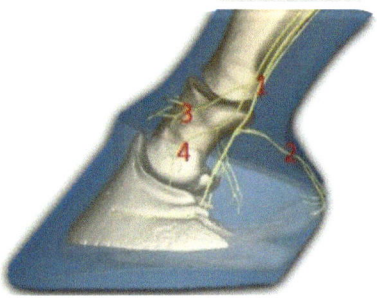

Nerves of the lower limb *

1. Lateral palmar digital nerve
2. Lateral ungular torus nerve
3. Dorsal digital nerve
4. Middle digital nerve

The dorsal digital nerve and middle digital nerve receive impulses from the coronary corium, extensor process of the coffin bone and the dorsal aspect of the coffin joint.

The palmar digital nerves receive impulses from the solar surface of the coffin bone, navicular bone, digital cushion and sole corium. There are also small peripheral nerves found within the soft tissue structures of the foot which are then transmitted to larger nerves and the central nervous system.

Ligaments of the lower limb

A ligament is a band of fibrous connective tissue that links two bones together at a joint.

Ligaments that are found either side of a joint are referred to as collateral ligaments which can stretch to allow joints to open on one side if the hoof and limb loads the ground unevenly.

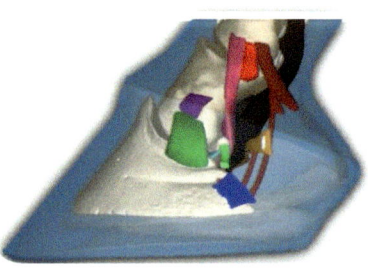

Ligaments of the lower limb * (Lateral view):

Dark Green – Lateral collateral ligament.

Dark blue – Lateral collateral chondroungal ligament.

Black – Distal Digital annular ligament.

White – Lateral chrondpulvine ligament.

Light green – Lateral chrondosesamoid ligament.

Purple – Lateral chondrocoronal ligament.

Pink – Lateral collateral sesamoidean ligament

The anatomy of the hoof

Dark yellow - Lateral cruciate chondroungal ligament.

Brown - Lateral chondroungalcomp ligament.

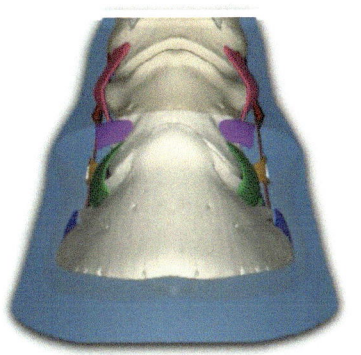

*The dorsal view showing the same ligaments from the lateral view on the opposite side of the joint and therefore classified as collateral ligaments. ***

Examination for lameness

Lameness is an indication of a structural or functional disorder in one or more limbs. It can be evident in the standing position but normally more noticeable during movement. Lameness can occur under these headings:

- Trauma.
- Congenital (from birth).
- Acquired abnormalities (marked deviations from normal).
- Infection.
- Metabolic compromises.
- Circulatory or neurological disorders.

The diagnosis of lameness requires a detailed knowledge of anatomy and physiology of the limb's movements with an appreciation for geometric design and subsequent forces.

Classification of lameness

Supporting limb lameness

This lameness occurs when the horse lands on the hoof and tries to shift weight off the limb as quickly as possible. Injury to bones, joints, soft tissue structures and motor nerves of the foot are considered to be associated with this type of lameness.

Swinging limb lameness

This lameness is evident when the limb is in motion. Injuries to the joint capsules, muscles, tendons, tendon sheaths or bursas are often associated with this type of lameness.

Mixed lameness

This is a combination of supporting and swinging limb lameness which can involve any of the structures mentioned above. The gait must be observed to establish which of the two types is the main factor in the lameness. There are some conditions that cause supporting limb lameness that may make the horse alter their gait to protect the foot they land on. This can sometimes lead to misdiagnosis of swinging limb lameness.

Compensatory lameness

This occurs when pain is found on a single limb or hoof and then leads to an uneven distribution of weight on other limbs. Lameness may then develop on a previously sound healthy limb due to increased stress and force from supporting the original lame limb.

Bibliography

Butler, D & Butler, J. (2004) *'The Principles of Horseshoeing (P3)'*, Doug Butler Enterprises: Colorado, USA.

Colles, C., Ware, R., & Hayes, J. (2022) *'Principles of Farriery'* The Crowood Press: Marlborough

Goody, P. C. (1976) *'Horse anatomy. A pictorial approach to equine structure'*, JA Allen: London

Hickman, J., & Humphrey, M. (1988) *'Hickman's farriery'* JA Allen: London

* Images adapted with kind permission from Effigos AG. Hoof Explorer

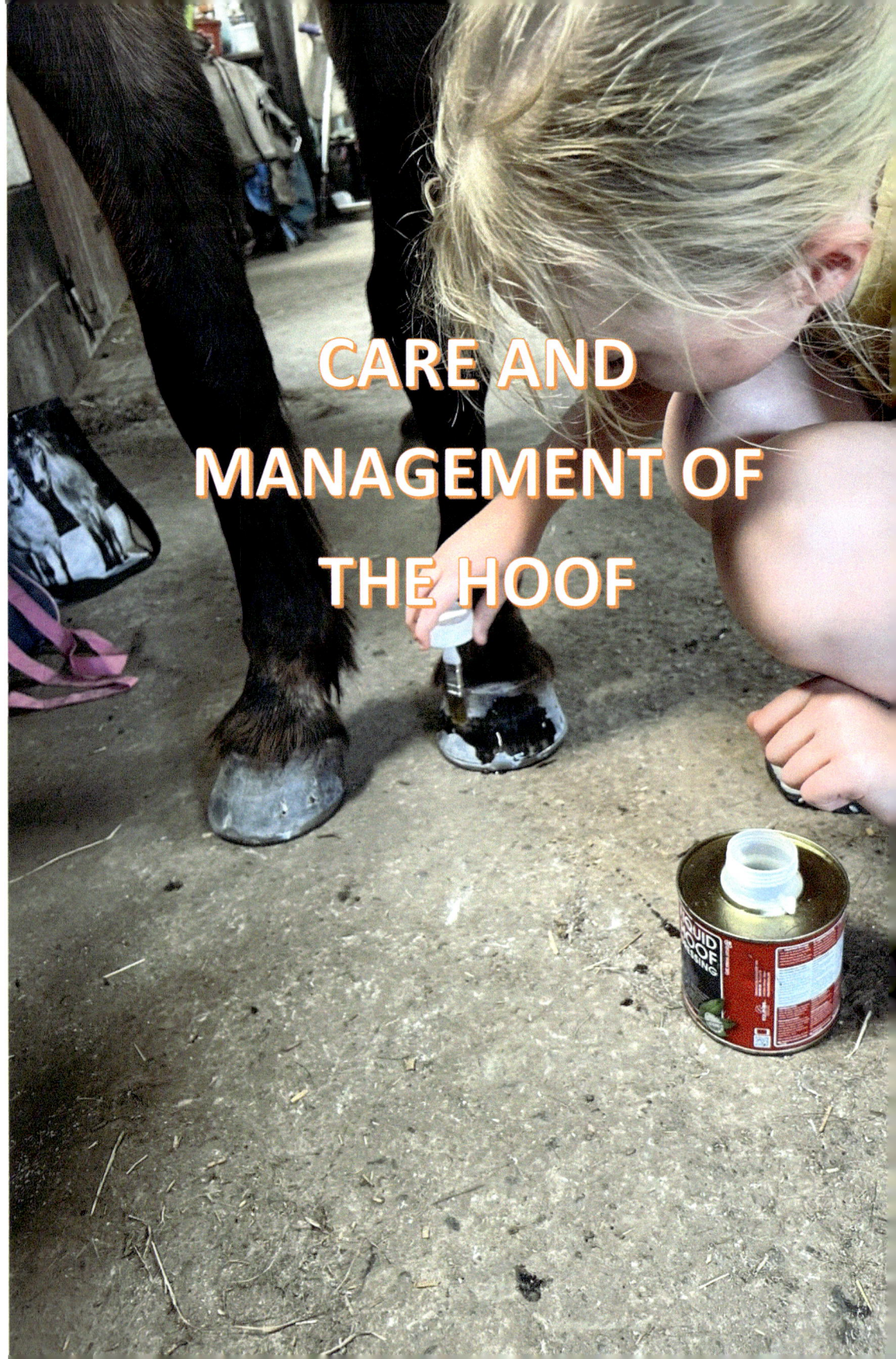

Chapter 2 - Care and management of the hoof

Presenting your horse for assessment

When presenting your horse for assessment by your farrier, vet or hoof care practitioner, it is recommended they are clean and dry with all four hooves picked out. This will help the person working on your horse to have a clear vision of the limbs and the horse's gait when being walked or trotted up. A secure tie up area on hard standing with cover is advisable for safe working conditions and to take shelter from adverse weather conditions.

In order to further provide a safe working environment, ensure the area is free from trip hazards or items that could easily blow over or get knocked by the horse being worked on (Fig. 2.1). Where possible, leave the horse's field companion in a nearby stable for company and avoid distributing bucket feeds to the rest of the stabled horses. If it is a hot day and flies are present, applying a fly repellent will help to keep the horse calm.

A fly rug can sometimes be used but it must be applied securely to reduce the chances of the practitioner being caught up in the rug whilst working on the horse. The above measures won't prevent all incidents but will help prevent the majority and result in a better standard of hoof care.

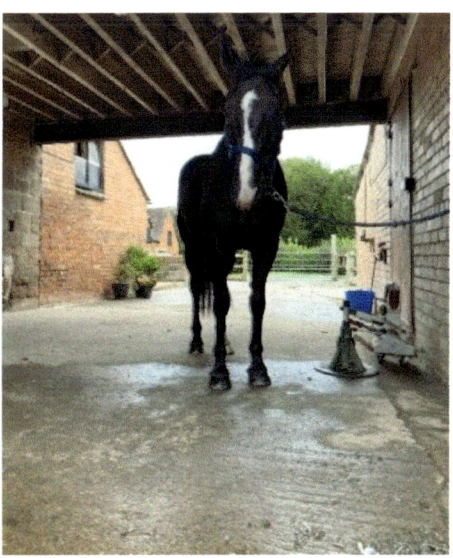

Fig. 2.1 An example of a safe working area with flat level concrete, cover from extreme weathers, allowing for air flow, free from clutter with a safe tie up to a strong wall.

Care and management of the hoof

Hoof first aid kit

When hoof emergencies arise, it is recommended to have a first aid kit present on the stable yard to minimise the damage caught as soon as possible. The list of recommended tools and products include:

- Farrier's nailing hammer
- Hoof buffer
- Shoe pullers
- Poultice kit (Animal intex, vet wrap, duct tape)
- Hoof boots appropriate to the size of your horse's hoof.
- Antiseptic spray

Removing a shoe in an emergency

A half lost shoe results in an emergency of greater urgency than if the shoe is lost entirely (Fig. 2.2). This is due to the possibility of a horse standing on a clip or a nail which could lead to an infection.

Before attempting to remove a shoe on a horse that is reluctant to weight bear, it is recommended to send a photo of the sole side of the hoof to either your farrier or vet who can advise whether it is safe to proceed if they cannot attend themselves.

This because some punctures may require a radiograph to evaluate the area of insertion and whether any vital structures have become effected.

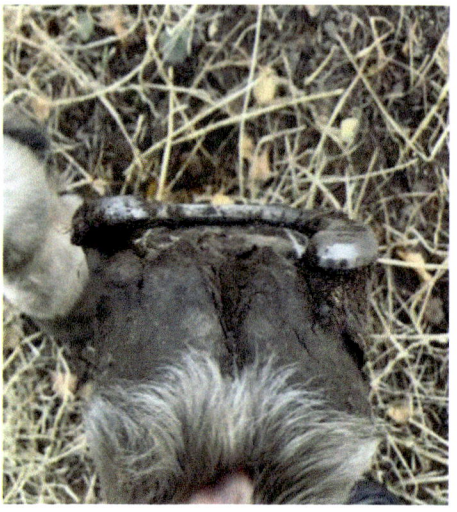

Fig. 2.2 A shoe that has lifted on one side whilst being fully secure on the opposite side.

Following this, ensure the area is free from clutter and any trip hazards so you can perform the shoe removal safely. Practice being able to hold your horse's front feet between your legs and having both hands free, this is essential for a successful shoe removal.

Pick out the sole side of the hoof using a hoof pick and repeat on the other 3 feet if possible but if the horse cannot bear weight on the affected hoof, this is not recommended. Then follow these procedures:

Care and management of the hoof

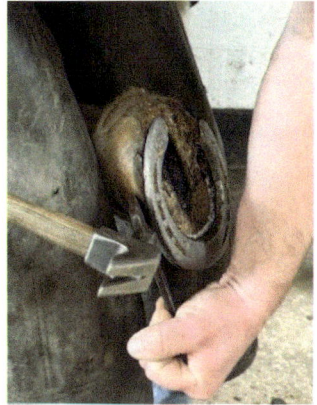

1. Using the hammer and buffer, directly blow the base of the clinches on the lateral (outside) of the hoof, working at a slight angle to get the lift of the base of the nail.

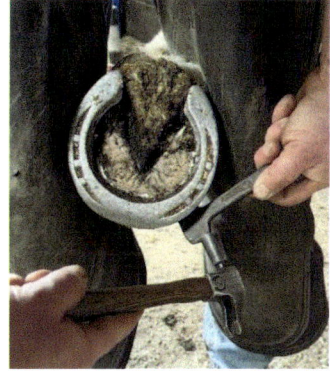

2. Place the hoof back on the ground if you require a rest at this point before repeating the same procedure on the medial (inside) side of the hoof.

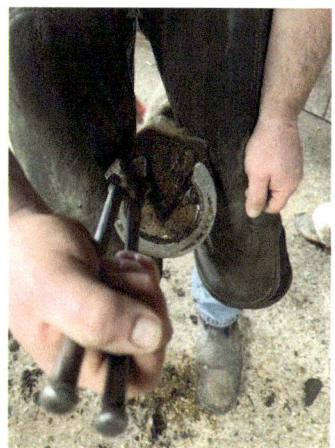

3. Place the shoe pullers under the heel of the lateral heel and close the reins together until the jaws touch. Then with both arms free, lever downwards in the direction of the bend of the shoe.

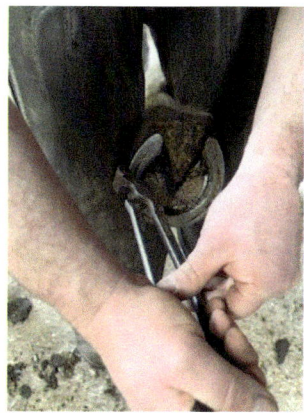

4. Move down in one inch increments, closing up the reins and levering down in the same way until you reach the nail hole closest to the toe.

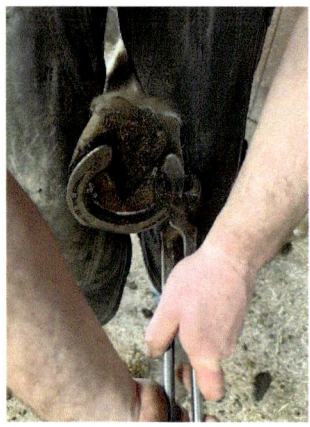

5. Switch to the medial branch and repeat the same procedure as the lateral branch until there is enough movement to pivot the toe of the shoe in either direction and the shoe comes away from the hoof.

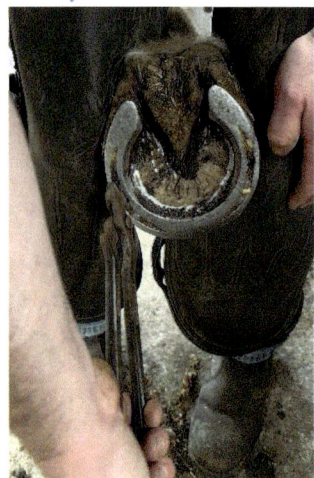

6. In a newly shod hoof, individual nails can be removed by following the same procedure of knocking up nail clenches and then using nail pullers to remove each nail. Remove one from every side until no nails are left in the hoof and the shoe can be lifted off by hand.

Neglected feet

When working with neglected feet, it must be stressed that a careful and thorough diagnostic approach is taken to prevent causing further suffering (Hemsworth et al. 2021). It is often the temptation to trim away excess hoof in order to make the horse more comfortable but without the use of radiographs, the position of the pedal bone and any internal damage or fracture cannot be determined (Fig. 2.3).

Diagnostic blood tests can also be performed at this stage to assess any hormonal pathology present. If the horse is nervous or unhandled, then it is advisable to have veterinary prescribed sedation administered to the horse in order to keep the farrier, owner and horse at a lower risk of injury.

Care and management of the hoof

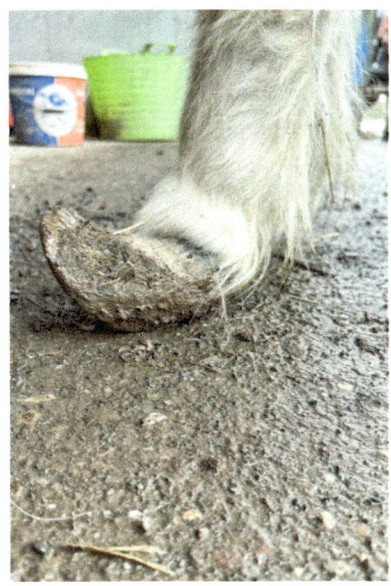

Fig. 2.3 An example of a pony whose hooves have overgrown leading to lameness and a difficulty in bearing weight on any limb.

Offer a soft mat for the opposite hoof to stand on whilst trimming if lameness is present and keep providing a rest period for horses that are new to the trimming process. There are some cases that would benefit from a gradual, weekly trim to normal hoof proportions rather than trying to achieve the ideal before trimming again in 6 weeks (Johns, 2014). This is more common in cases with excessively long toes that have put a large strain on the suspensory apparatus and associated ligaments.

Preventative measures to help avoid emergencies

There are many cases where injury or trauma can be avoided with simple changes. Whilst this won't solve every issue, they are worth considering as implementing as part of the daily routine.

Pick out feet daily

This may sound simple but daily picking out of feet when brought in from a field can help prevent sole pressure from hard dirt pressing against the sole and potentially leading to a bruise (Fig. 2.4).

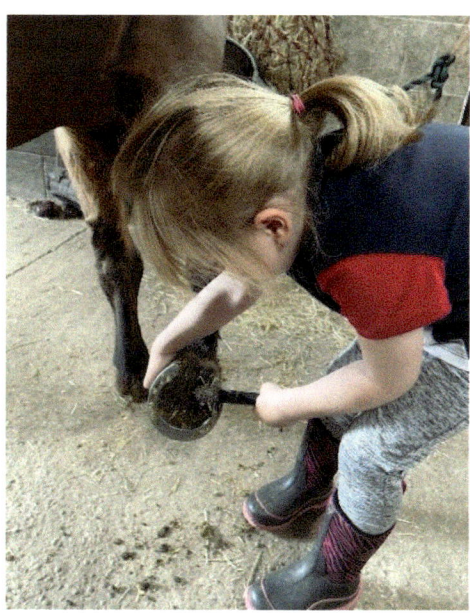

Fig. 2.4 A daily routine of picking out feet can identify any potential issues and stop them becoming major problems.

Drying feet

During the winter months, it is often tempting to cold hose down muddy feet but this can lead to a weakening of the defences of the lower limb with potential mud fever or bacterial infections of the hoof. It is much more preferable to towel dry muddy hooves and legs with the option of leg wraps for turnout providing the horse isn't sensitive skinned.

Punctured sole from a nail

There could also be a foreign body such as a nail or screw that has punctured the sole or frog (Fig. 2.5). If this has occurred, it is strongly advised that it is not removed before being assessed by a vet or farrier due to the risk of sensitive structures being damaged and an infection developing (Steckel et al. 1990).

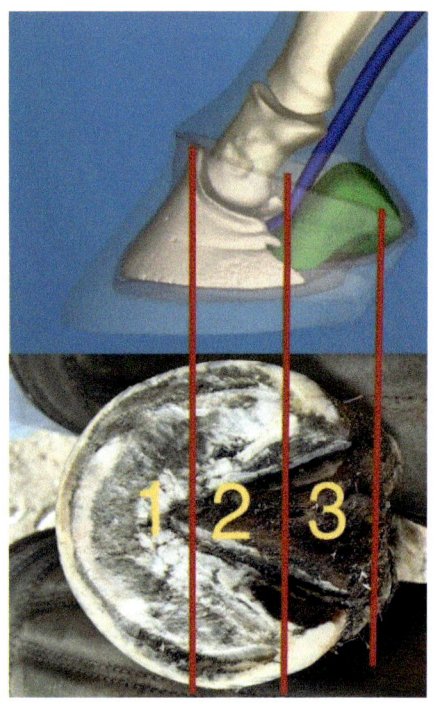

Fig. 2.5 The three areas of sole puncture. Although every puncture requires immediate attention, area 2 is the most serious due to the potential of the navicular bursa and deep digital flexor tendon being damaged. Area 3 is the least serious due to the digital cushion taking up most of the area although an infection is still possible. *

Whilst it is tempting to remove an object, it can create an infection that in some cases can be fatal. It is best advised to note the likely depth of penetration of the nail/screw and take a photo using your phone to send to your farrier or vet (Fig. 2.6). Using a spare lost shoe, tape this to the existing shoe and wrap the hoof as if you were poulticing, this will help to prevent the object being pushed further into the sole and keep the horse on box rest until a vet has visited.

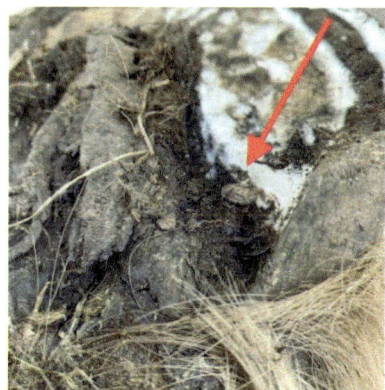

Fig. 2.6 A nail that has penetrated through the collateral groove of the frog.

Radiography can then take place to determine the depth of penetration and whether a referral to a hospital is required to perform surgery and remove all damaged hoof and repair soft tissue damage (Barr, 2022). If this were to happen, a hospital plate shoe can be applied to seal the hoof completely and allow for daily treatment post surgery until the cavity has grown out.

It must be stressed that the vast majority of hoof punctures aren't life threatening but careful steps taken in the early stages can provide a greater chance of success in the later stages.

Checking for an increased pulse

There may be times when a horse is lame, that an increased digital pulse to the lower limb can be detected. This is useful for helping detect lameness such as a solar abscess, laminitis, or trauma. Simply place your finger and thumb in the hollow just above the fetlock and if a throbbing is noticed, then the horse has an increased pulse that warrants further investigation (Fig. 2.7).

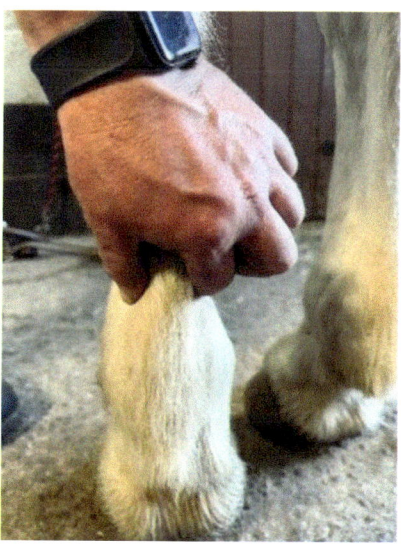

Fig. 2.7 Placing your index finger and thumb with pressure in the hollow just above the fetlock can help to detect an increased pulse to the hoof.

The use of overreach boots

Overreach boots are fitted around the pastern to cover and protect the rear of the hoof in its entirety. This is to offer protection in this area from a hind hoof collision and help prevent shoe loss. The boot should cover the entirety of the rear of the hoof and heel bulbs to fit correctly (Fig. 2.8).

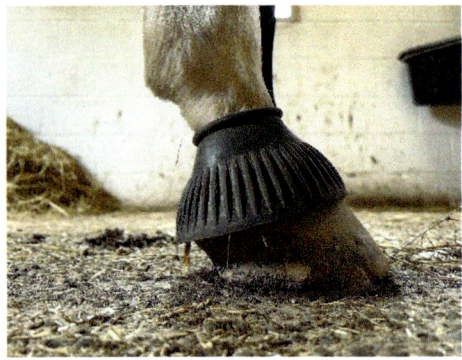

Fig. 2.8 An example of an overreach boot that is too small in depth and doesn't fully protect the rear of the hoof.

Due to the shape of the pastern in some horses, particularly the sport horse types with little hair, they can ride up and expose the heels during trot or canter. In order to overcome this, a sausage boot can be fitted above the overreach boot to prevent it riding up and offer full time protection (Fig. 2.9).

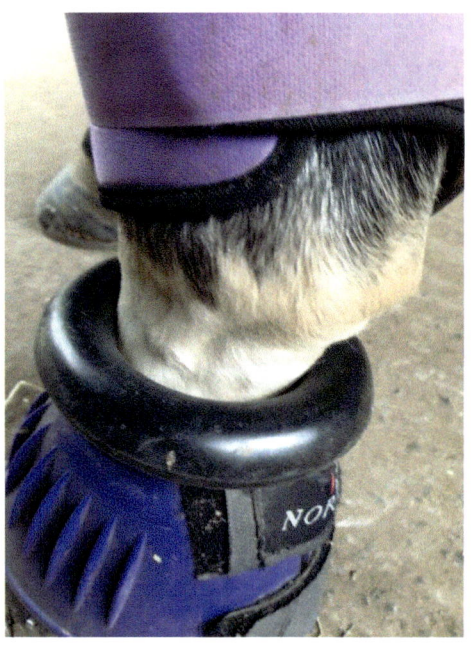

Fig. 2.9 A sausage boot fitted above an overreach boot can prevent the boot from rising on horses with skinny pasterns offering protection when the horse is trotting or cantering.

There can be incidents where the rim of the overreach boot rubs the heel bulbs and coronary band, particularly if there is a fleece lining that is holding a lot of moisture (Fig. 2.10). Therefore, it is important to remove the boots during time spent in the stable or when protection is less required. Check to ensure the rim of the boot is not too tight, if rubbing persists then a layer of Vaseline applied to the rim of the boot can help to limit the level of friction.

Care and management of the hoof

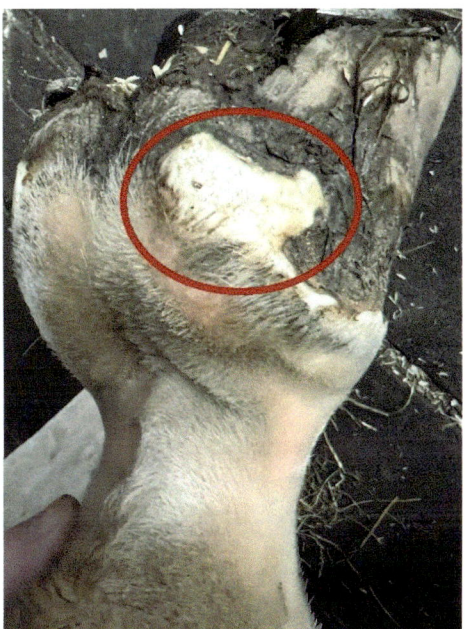

Fig. 2.10 An example of rubbing at the heel bulbs from long term use of overreach boots.

Warming up correctly

Whilst the purpose of this book is to offer solutions on hoofcare, the benefits of correct riding and warming up should be considered to prevent injury to the soft tissues or a potential interference injury resulting in time off work (Fig. 2.11). A good amount of time spent walking and encouraging stretching at the beginning and end of a schooling session is advised along with a variety of work on different surfaces during the week. Horses that have just come in from the field to be ridden will require less warming up than those who have been kept in a stable overnight. A well warmed up horse is less likely to trip or have limbs colliding as well as giving the ligaments of the lower limb the elastic strength they need.

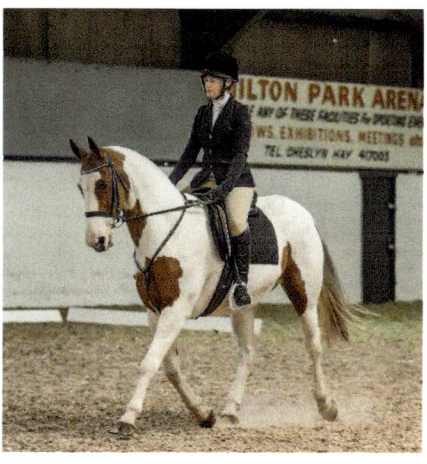

Fig. 2.11 A horse warmed up correctly is less likely to encounter performance issues.

Applying hoof dressing

As the hoof hardens in response to a dry and hard environment, the fracture point lowers so it can break up quite easily. Whilst there is no scientific proof that applying hoof dressing alters the moisture content of the inner hoof, it is the author's opinion that regular hoof dressing during dry spells can lead to healthier feet (Fig. 2.12).

Care and management of the hoof

This is even the case if there are already chipped up pieces of hoof as when the hooves are trimmed back to a functional proportion, the hoof above the chipping is of a more flexible structure and is capable of working on a harder surface.

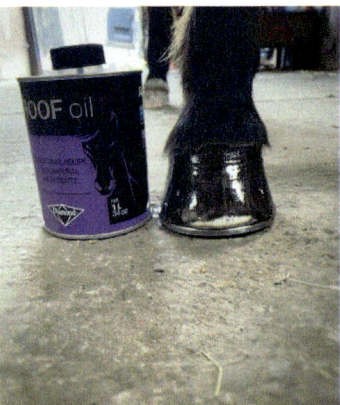

Fig. 2.12 A daily coating of hoof dressing can help prevent the external surface of the hoof wall from fractures and help to maintain flexibility.

Removing unsuitable fencing

It is important to consider the type of fencing that your horses are turned out within. A loose or unstable fence could lead to a horse escaping or creating an injury during the process. Sheep wire is a type of fencing that should be avoided with horses due to the shape of the wire squares being perfectly sized to get a hoof trapped in, leading to either shoe loss or partial loss of the heel bulb (Fig. 2.13).

Whilst the benefits of this type of fencing can be seen for keeping dogs out, consider using a strip of electric fence a yard away from the fencing so that the horses are kept safe from becoming tangled up. The same can be said for barbed wire with the risk of severe injury if a horse runs through it and getting wrapped around a leg.

The ideal type of fencing should be a post and rail wooden fence or electric tape as there is far less risk of an injury occurring.

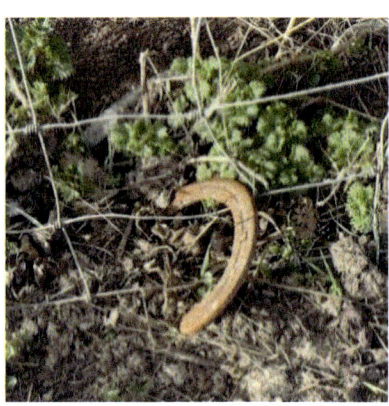

Fig. 2.13 A lost shoe from a horse getting caught in sheep wire fencing.

Finding lost shoes

Whilst lost shoes are a great source of frustration for owners and farriers, it is important that lost shoes are located in order to reduce the risk of sole punctures. The use of a metal detector can help to locate shoes in deeper mud. Although it is desirable to locate every nail, as long as the shoe is found a couple of missing nails will most likely sink in the mud without causing damage. The shoe can hold the nails in an upright position making it easier to penetrate the sole. The heels of the shoe can also puncture the sole if struck into at the wrong angle (Fig. 2.14).

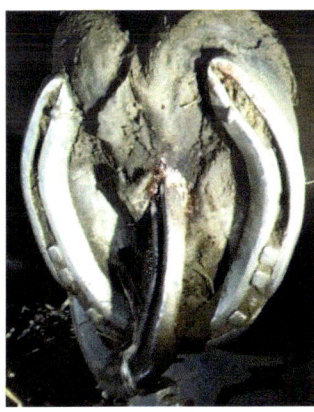

Fig. 2.14 An example of a lost shoe that has punctured the frog resulting in a complicated injury that requires immediate veterinary attention. Photo credit: Mark Aikens

Hoof management of horses on box rest

If a horse must stay on box rest for a period of time, it is advisable to maintain the bedding as clean as possible to reduce the risk of thrush and other infections developing. Regular picking out and applying anti fungal clay to the sole and frog will help to reduce the bacteria present. A regular hoof trimming cycle if the pathology allows, can help detect any issues early on.

Snow packed in the hoof

When there is excessive snowfall there can be a build up of snow in the sole and frog, especially if the horse is shod (Fig. 2.15). Therefore, it is important to provide regular picking out of the hooves if the horse lives out and encourage them into a shelter by placing hay there. There is limited evidence to suggest that painting the sole with Vaseline can help prevent the snow from sticking to the hoof, often it is better to keep the horse on box rest for a couple of days if snowfall is forecast to continue.

However, if the horse is kept in a part of the world where snowfall lasts for months, the application of snow pads can help to push out excess snow and prevent sole pressure. The shoes may also require extra traction with the application of studs to help prevent slipping.

Care and management of the hoof

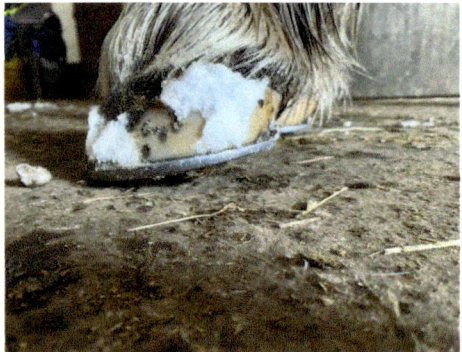

Fig. 2.15 A hoof that is unable to contact the ground due to excessive snow packed in the sole.

The use of track systems

There has been an uptake in the use of track systems over the last few years which involve fencing off and creating a track in a large field involving a variety of surfaces for the horse to walk over (Hampson et al. 2010). This can be used for both shod and unshod horses. The theory behind this is to encourage movement, increase strength of the hoof, build soft tissue within the hoof and provide a grassless diet whereby the horse's nutritional intake can be controlled by hay and mineral supplementation.

There are numerous designs aimed at increased movement of a population of horses (Fig. 2.16).

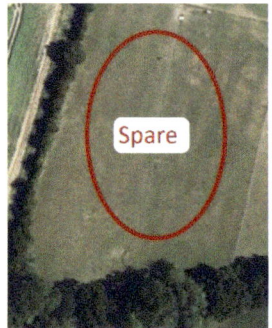
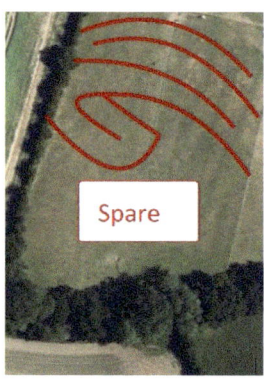
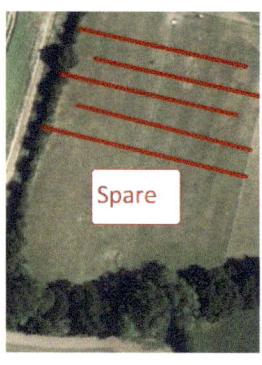

Fig. 2.16 An example of various track system designs. The areas labelled "spare" are not grazed, often they are cut for hay.

Care and management of the hoof

Horses tend to live in herds on a track system and are kept out permanently. There are clear benefits for the enrichment of the horse and for those horses that tend to "stiffen up" from being kept in along with horses that are recovering from a case of laminitis.

However, this style of management may not be suitable for competition horses that are clipped or at risk from injury from another horse. There also must be consideration of the intake of minerals such as iron from the soils of these grassless environments which can invoke an inflammatory response in the horse.

Therefore, a thorough assessment of soil, grass and hay analysis should be performed before considering this option.

Barefoot versus shod

The barefoot versus shod debate has been going on for decades if not centuries. There are many facets and situations where either is appropriate with scientific studies proving the credibility of both methods. It is the opinion of the author that the debate should be barefoot versus protection due to the range of high quality hoof boots, composite shoes and pads combined with steel shoes now available.

Indeed, the traditional open heel shoe is now less prevalent than ever due to the issues with peripheral loading of the hoof that a standard shoe provides. This is more noticeable in low heeled horses where the frog and heel bulbs begin to prolapse through the centre of the shoe (Malone & Davies, 2019).

Due to the prolapse of the frog and heel bulbs, there are a wide range of frog support pads available to prevent this occurring although the frog may not have a rigid hardness due to the pad making the structure soft and deformable.

There has been a marked change in the last 25 years in the way horses have been managed and trained. Due to the introduction and availability of synthetic arena surfaces, horses are now in work all year round rather than having a winter break due to the grass arenas being too wet to ride in. This has resulted in horses being shod all year round rather than having a few months barefoot and being turned out for winter grazing and having access to biodiversity in their forage.

It is the author's opinion that if the horse requires shoes, then there are many advantages to also having a rest period of four months of the year where the horse is barefoot. This is much more achievable in the winter with softer ground and it being easier to control the sugar levels in the diet with hay and grain feed.

We do have to recognise the limits that our horses can be ridden for or competed at, and these may not match our ambitions. It is recommended that each horse is assessed fully on their management, conformation and fitness levels prior to commencement of hoofcare whether they are shod or barefoot.

Hoof boots

Hoof boots are a good alternative to provide suitable protection that can be removed when not riding or walking on abrasive surfaces. Taking a measure of the length and width of the solear surface of the hoof will allow the horse owner to find a suitable size of hoof boot in a design that suits their horse (Fig. 2.17 and 2.18). The standard of hoof boot has improved considerably over the years with much lighter and efficient designs for a variety of disciplines.

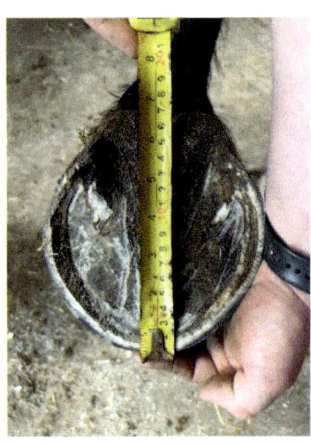

Fig. 2.17 Measuring the hoof width across the widest part.

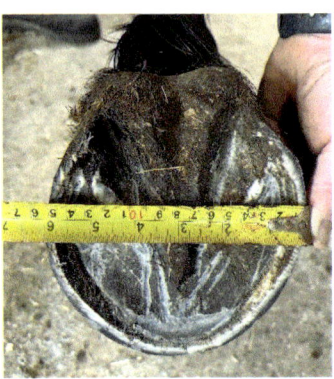

Fig. 2.18 Measuring the length of the hoof from the toe to point at which the heels bisect.

When checking the fit of your hoof boot, you should be able to push your finger between the straps at the heel and the heel bulbs. There should be a small gap between the top of the hoof boot and the coronary band to prevent rubbing. Then pick up the hoof and see if you can wiggle the boot in either direction before walking the horse away and back to ensure the boot doesn't twist or move on the hoof (Fig. 2.19). If the turnout conditions are wet, then only use the boots when the horse is walking across hard and abrasive surfaces where protection is more required. If the horse is stabled for a prolonged period, then boots won't be required during this time due to the bedding providing adequate comfort.

One of the disadvantages to hoof boots is the effect of rubbing at the coronary band and heel bulbs which can lead to soreness. If this occurs, then applying a thin layer of Vaseline to the area can reduce the effects of the boot rubbing. Also consider the rules for competing with hoof boots as British Dressage do not allow horses to compete with more than 50% of any hoof covered by any material (British Dressage Tack & Equipment, 2023).

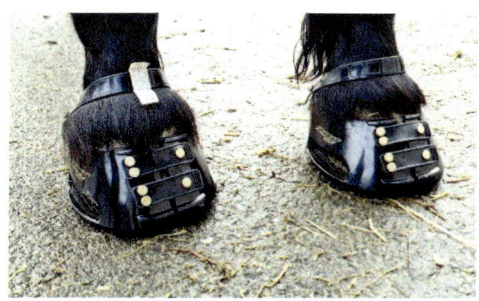

Fig. 2.19 A pair of boots fitted to hooves that are maintained barefoot.

The role of composite shoes

Composite shoes are now becoming more commonplace in hoof care as they offer greater sole protection and frog engagement than open heeled steel shoes. In some cases of horses with degenerative joint disease, the reduction of concussion from the plastic material with the ground compared to steel is seen as advantageous (Syem et al. 2022). The lightweight material that can flex with the ground can also help to replicate the functionality of the barefoot hoof (Fig. 2.20).

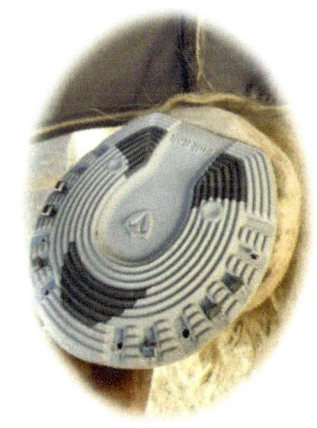

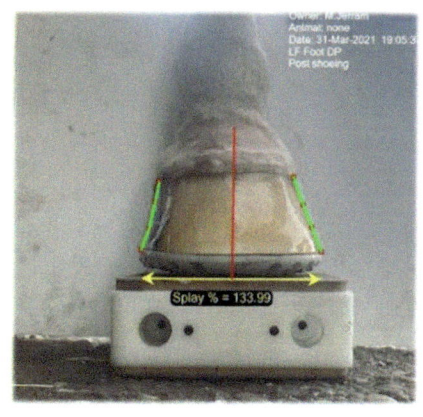

Fig. 2.20 A full roll composite shoe applied with nails. The rolling edges make it easier for horses to turn.

The design of these shoes allow for easy modification should any bevelling be required to the outer edge and help reduce leverage when turning (Fig. 2.21). There are some downfalls to these applications such as the inability to gain access to the frog area for cleaning, so it is advised that an anti fungal clay is applied heavily first to reduce the chances of bacteria forming.

concussion and vibration from a hard road surface (Fig. 2.22). Quite often, these are applied to carriage horses that are working in town centres to help limit the noise from shod hooves. The rubber shoes provide less traction on grass however, so the horse's expected work should be considered before application.

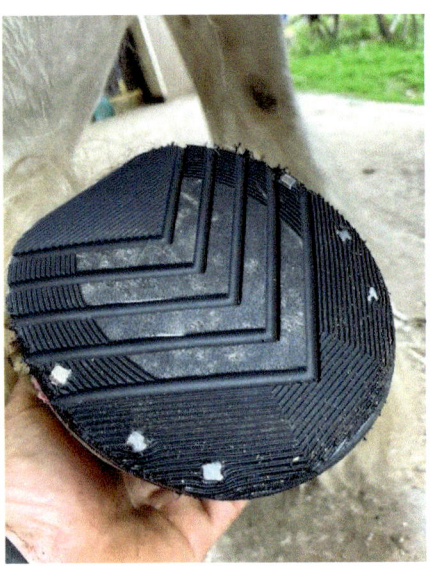

Fig. 2.21 A pair of rocker composite shoes helping a horse with arthritic changes to the coffin joint.

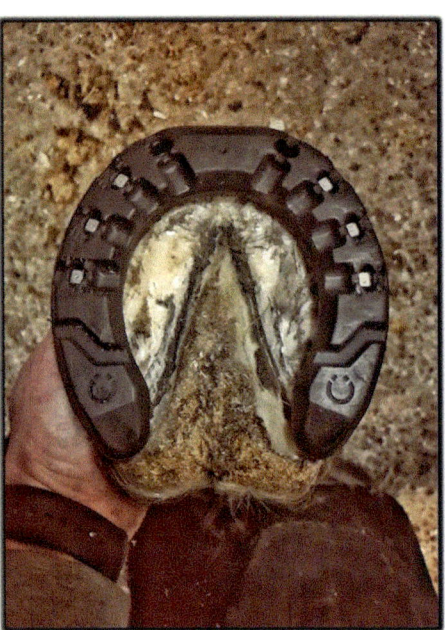

Fig. 2.22 A rubber shoe applied to a horse that does a lot of road work.

Rubber shoes

Rubber shoes have a steel core to allow for shaping but maintain their form throughout the shoeing cycle as a result. They are nailed in the same fashion as a steel shoe and are useful for reducing

Glue on composite shoes

Glue on composite shoes tend not to have a steel core so the application can flex with the natural function of the hoof (Fig. 2.23). The shoes can be applied with or without frog support depending on the functionality of the hoof and of any pathology is present. The disadvantage of using glue applications is the increased risk of bacteria forming under the glue on tabs and degenerating hoof wall quality along with the possibility of hoof contraction.

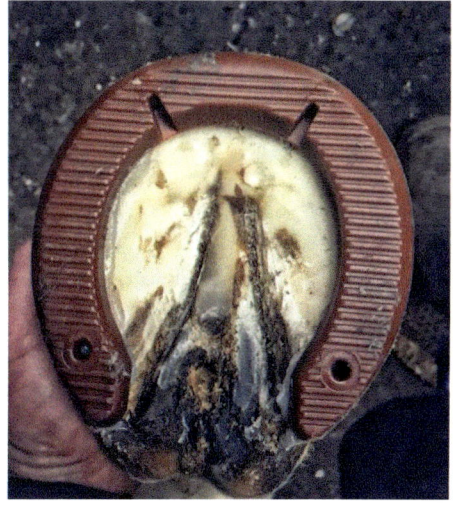

Fig. 2.23 A glue on urethane shoe applied to a horse with navicular syndrome that benefitted from flexible hoof protection.

Arena surfaces and the hoof

There are now a variety of artificial surfaces that horses can work and compete on with the number of grass arenas declining. As these artificial surfaces are of different densities and hardness, they can have a notable effect on the interaction with the hoof and limb. Common arena surfaces include, silca sand, rubber, carpet fibre or a mixture of materials.

As the hoof lands, it stops and slides forwards and downwards into the surface and the bones collide within the lower limb and hoof. Concussion is absorbed and distributed to the ground and leg. During the stance phase, the whole hoof is stationary carrying the horse's bodyweight into the surface (Holt et al. 2014). The fetlock, flexor tendons and suspensory ligament create a shock absorption effect. The loading force depends upon movements such as collection or landing from a jump. The toe then rolls into the surface to allow breakover of the hoof and limb to begin with propulsion.

An ideal arena surface allows horses to move efficiently through these phases. The surface should be able to minimise concussion, absorb shock, provide support and return energy. In order to achieve this the surface should have characteristics such as firmness, cushioning, cupping, rebound and grip.

Firmness

Firmness refers to the support and shock force distribution during the landing phase of the stride. A surface that is too firm will increase concussion to the joints of the lower limb and hoof. A surface that is lacking in firmness reduces support to the ascending limb and puts

Care and management of the hoof

tension on tendons and ligaments along with causing fatigue. The ideal surface dissipates concussion equally during the landing phase (Fig. 2.24).

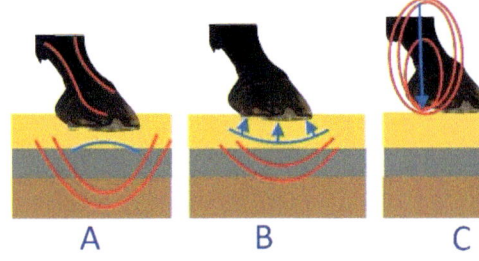

Fig. 2.25 Arena surface that is too soft and deep (A), Ideal (B) and too compact (C).

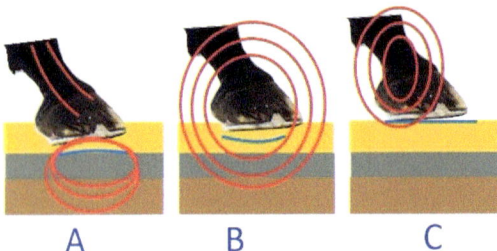

Fig. 2.24 An arena surface that is too soft (A), Ideal (B) and too hard (C).

Cushioning

Cushioning is how the arena layers dampen shock during the stance phase. If the surface is too compact, it lacks cushion and reduces stress and shock relief. As a result, the hoof becomes excessively loaded with weight. However, if the surface is too soft and deep, it will shift under foot and the horse will have to work harder for support and energy. This increases the risk of inflammation to the soft tissues of the hoof and lower limb. The ideal surface will dampen shock efficiently with minimal stress to the hoof and limb (Fig. 2.25).

Cupping

Cupping is the act of supporting the sole and pedal bone when the horse is in the stance phase and the frog becomes stimulated for circulation. A surface that is too compact will hinder hoof mechanism and create a lack of blood flow through smaller veins. A soft surface will cup under the foot but may result in a lack of resistance and pressure under the frog. The ideal surface will cup into the sole and collateral grooves, will support weight evenly and stimulate the frog with pressure (fig. 2.26).

Care and management of the hoof

Rebound

Rebound is the resiliency of the surface to return to its original form and therefore return energy to the horse. A surface that is too stiff will rebound too quickly so the shock and vibrations will become absorbed by the horse. However, an arena surface that is too deep will rebound too slowly and increases the amount of energy required by the horse's tendons and ligaments. An ideal surface will return energy to the horse equally whilst minimizing the amount of vibration (fig. 2.27).

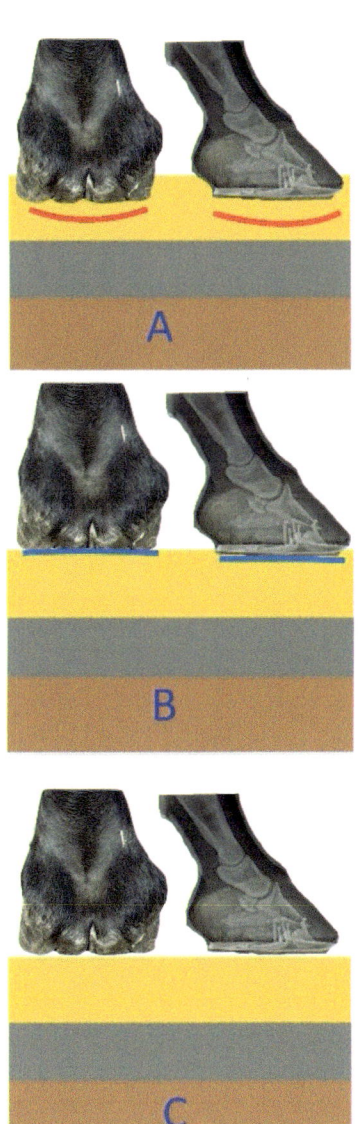

Fig. 2.26 Arena effects on cupping of the hoof – Too soft (A), Ideal (B) and too compact (C).

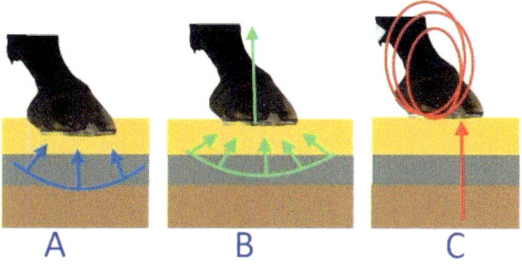

Fig. 2.27 Types of rebound on an arena surface – Too deep (A), Ideal (B) and too stiff (C).

Grip

Grip aids in absorbing shock during the landing phase whilst also providing support and traction during breakover and on turns. A surface that is too tight will stop the foot too quickly and therefore the stride becomes restricted. This increases the likelihood of injury to

Care and management of the hoof

joint surfaces. A surface that is too slippery will provide too much hoof slide and decreased propulsion (Fig. 2.28) As a consequence, this can lower the horse's confidence and performance. The ideal surface will allow the hoof to glide, stopping just enough to allowing the hoof to absorb impact forces. The tightness of the surface must allow the horse to have stability during breakover (Fig. 2.29).

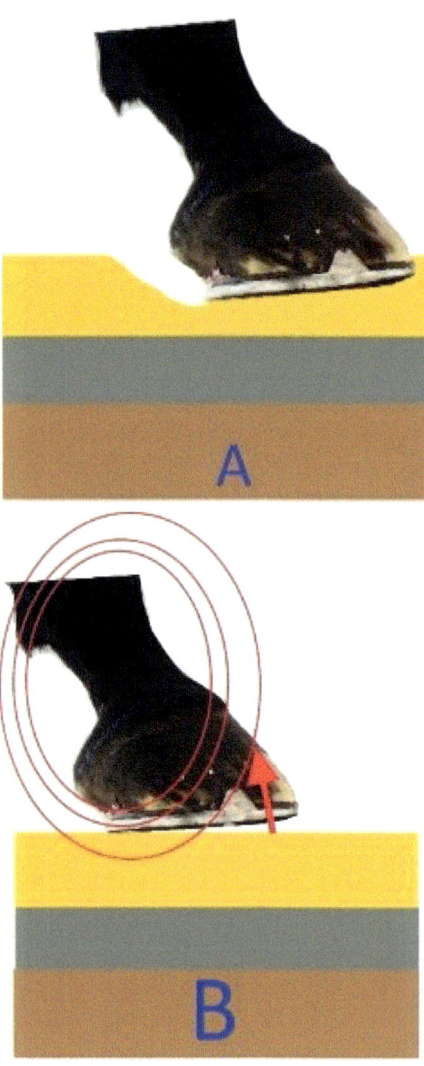

Fig. 2.28 The landing phase on an arena that is too slippery (A) and too tight (B)

Care and management of the hoof

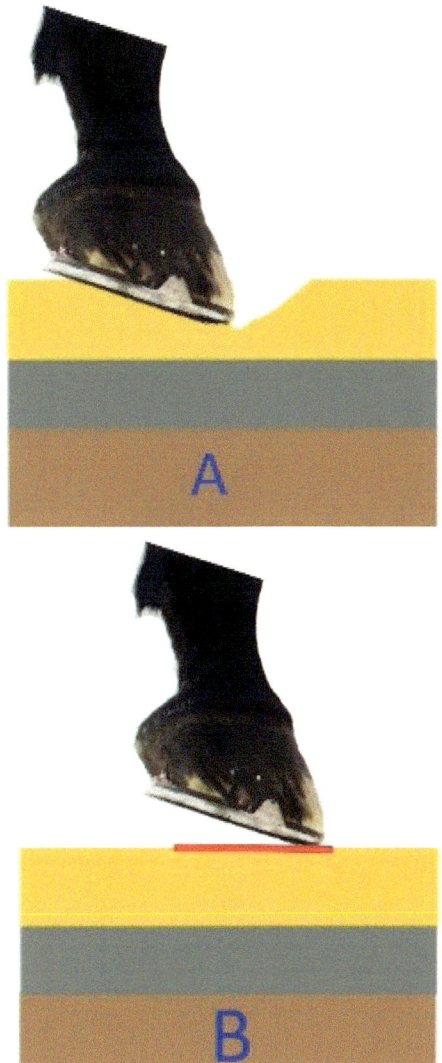

The arena must be well maintained to provide a quality surface for the horse to work on and prevent injury. This includes regular rolling, harrowing, and watering when required.

Fig. 2.29 The breakover phase on an arena that is too slippery (A) and too tight (B).

References

Barr, E. (2022) 'Surgery of the equine hoof: a review' *UK-Vet Equine*, Vol. *6*, No.4, pp 163-166.

British Dressage Tack & Equipment (2023) Available at: https://www.britishdressage.co.uk/media/6112/approved-tack-equipment-guide-2022-july.pdf (Accessed: 04 August 2023).

Hampson, B. A., Morton, J. M., Mills, P. C., Trotter, M. G., Lamb, D. W., & Pollitt, C. C. (2010) 'Monitoring distances travelled by horses using GPS tracking collars' *Australian Veterinary Journal*, Vol.*88*, No.5, pp 176-181.

Hemsworth, L. M., Jongman, E. C., & Coleman, G. J. (2021) 'The Human–Horse Relationship: Identifying the Antecedents of Horse Owner Attitudes towards Horse Husbandry and Management Behaviour' *Animals*, Vol.*11*, No.2 pp 278-284.

Holt, D., Northrop, A., Martin, J., Daggett, A., & Hobbs, S. (2014) 'What do riders want from an arena surface?' *Equine Veterinary Journal*, Vol. *46*, pp 41-42.

Johns, I. (2014) 'Veterinary management of starved and neglected horses' *In Practice*, Vol. 36, No.3, pp 144-152.

Malone, S. R., & Davies, H. M. (2019) 'Changes in hoof shape during a seven-week period when horses were shod versus barefoot' *Animals*, Vol. *9*, No.12, pp 1017-1022.

Steckel, R. R., Fessler, J. F., & Huston, L. C. (1990) 'Deep puncture wounds of the equine hoof: a review of 50 cases' In *Proceedings of the Annual Convention of the American Association of Equine Practitioners*, Vol. 35, pp. 167-176.

Syam, B., Muttaqin, M., Tantono, J., Eddo, E., & Sandry, F. (2022) 'The Design And Responses Of Horses On Polimeric Composite Horseshoes' *Jurnal Sistem Teknik Industri*, Vol. *24*, No.2, pp 273-279.

* Images adapted with kind permission from Effigos AG. Hoof Explorer

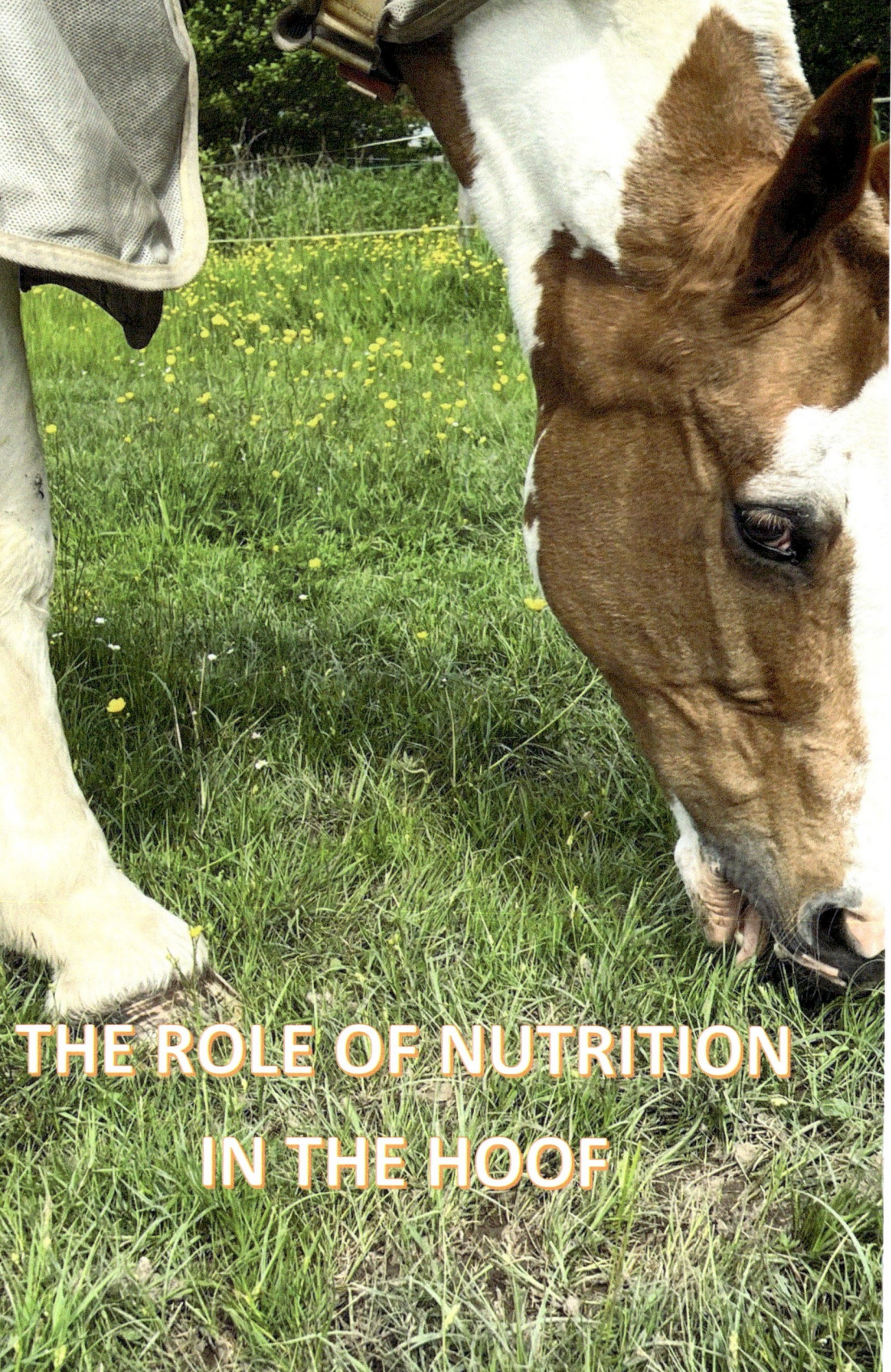

Chapter 3 – The role of nutrition in the hoof

Introduction

Although it would be impossible to deliver the total nutrition requirements of the horse's hoof in one section of this book, an introduction is provided to cover the essentials with an emphasis that each horse's requirements are unique, and that a thorough analysis should be performed prior to supplementation or any changes.

The quality of the hoof is dependent on a combination of endogenous and exogenous factors. The endogenous factors that influence hoof quality include chemical composition, stratum structure, the levels of intercellular fluid in addition to the amount and arrangement of cells. When it comes to the exogenous factors, feral horses have a major advantage over domesticated horses when it comes to their diet. This is due to the fact they get to travel over a larger area with greater exposure to a range of exogenous factors such as differing soil types, gradients and plant biodiversity.

The nutrient composition of the hoof wall is made up of 94% protein/amino acids with 3% of fat/oils. The remaining 3% is made up of trace minerals and vitamins such as sulphur, calcium, zinc, copper, selenium, vitamin A, vitamin B and Vitamin E.

Domesticated horses often eat the same feed and hay type every day with their turnout areas offering less plant variety than the feral horse have access to. The mineral profiles of iron, copper, zinc, manganese and selenium are likely to be similar due to the plants that are growing in the same soil.

Horses are able to interconvert fats, carbohydrates and amino acids (the building blocks of protein). They can increase the active absorption of minerals and are equipped with mechanisms to excrete excessive amounts of mineral except iron. However, not all amino and fatty acids can be manufactured. They are deemed to be essential and is complicated by the fact that minerals compete for absorption in the intestines.

The reason nutritional deficiencies show up in the hoof is because of the metabolically active tissue found in the hoof wall. The hoof becomes worn away and has to be replaced constantly. If the hoof is lacking one or more of the nutrients, then the quality of the hoof will suffer. All of the key nutrients must be

The role of nutrition in the hoof

present in correct amounts. An excess of a nutrient is just as harmful as a deficiency as they may crowd out and block nutrients that are in low concentration. The best way to avoid this is to ensure that the horse's hay and pasture have been analysed so that only the required nutrients are supplemented and therefore create a balanced diet.

Hay diet

The type and quantity of hay is vitally important for overall equine health including hoof health. It is important that hay is cut at the optimum nutrient levels. The moisture level of the species should be a maximum of 15% when cut for hay. Hay loses vitamins quickly, so feed/balancers are often required. This is especially important during the winter when there is less grass available or for horses that are grass affected. Grass hay with combined values for Water Soluble Carbohydrates (WSC) and starch below 10% is ideal for most horses.

Timothy hay

Timothy hay was one of the first grasses grown specifically for horse hay as it has a low to moderate calorie content and is a rich source of fibre. Timothy is quite a hardy grass and is good for soil health. The water soluble carbohydrates are high when the plant is young and can be in excess of 30% in early spring compared to 15% in late spring and 10% in late summer. The main drawback is the availability due to the significant amount of water required to grow the crop.

Cocksfoot

Cocksfoot is less palatable than other grasses and is a hard wearing grass that regrows quickly after cutting. Cocksfoot has a high protein content of up to 30% where a horse requires a daily intake of around 16%. The protein content does drop to around 10% when the plant is mature.

Fescues

Although there are over 450 different fescues, the ones most commonly seen in horse paddocks are meadow fescue, tall fescue and red fescue.

Meadow fescue is palatable throughout the growing stages and tends to head later in the year but can be sensitive to drought conditions.

Tall fescue grows early in the season but is considered unpalatable and therefore is better suited to hay than grazing. There is a potential of a mycotoxin risk if there is too much tall fescue in a grazing lay.

Red fescue is common in all grazing pastures and is a relatively slow growing and stress tolerant grass that has medium palatability. It will grow in all but the most acidic or water logged soils.

The role of nutrition in the hoof

Meadow hay

Meadow hay forms a soft texture that is easily consumed by horses with minimal waste. Meadow hay contains a higher calorie content than Timothy hay whilst maintaining similar levels of calcium and phosphorus.

Ryegrass hay

Ryegrass hay, sometimes referred to as perennial ryegrass, contains a higher level of WSC with an estimation of up to 35% that will remain high all season. Ryegrass is very palatable and quite hardy, so it recovers well from cutting in a variety of environments. However, it tends to make poor quality hay so is instead produced as Ryelage.

Haylage

Haylage is cut at optimised nutrient levels to a moisture content of 60% and then wrapped in plastic. The principle of this is to convert sugars to lactic acid by fermentation with anaerobic conditions required for the desirable fermentation of haylage to occur. The conversion to lactic acid allows the pH content to drop to between 4.8 and 5.8 which helps to prevent the production of mycotoxins and mould. Haylage will contain higher levels of digestible energy and protein than hay.

Haylage is cut before hay and as it is less mature contains higher levels of WSC but cannot be soaked to reduce sugars so is therefore less suitable for horses at risk of laminitis (Rueda-Carrillo et al. 2022).

Safe hay feeding for overweight horses

Hay should be fed at 1.5% of the horse's bodyweight with the weight of the hay based on dry hay before soaking using a scale with a hook to measure the weight of the haynet. Soaking the hay will reduce the sugars to an average of 5% by a process of soaking in hot water for half an hour before an hour soaked in cold water. Do not exceed this time as vital nutrients can be leached from the hay and a balancer would be required to replace those lost nutrients.

Hay analysis

A hay analysis will report the composition of the hay and the percentile of differing factors that will determine the effects of the diet (Fig. 3.1). The hay sample will be reported as sampled (these records nutrients in their natural state including moisture) or dry matter (nutrients with the moisture removed). It is recommended that the dry matter column is used as it creates a direct comparison of nutrients across different feeds and can simplify the ration balancing process. Also consider the source of the analysis as many are calculated for cattle rather than horses so it is advisable to obtain an equine specific forage analysis.

The role of nutrition in the hoof

	Results			
% Moisture	79.3			
% Dry Matter	20.7			
	As Sampled		Dry Matter	
Digestible Energy (DE), Mcal/kg		.47		2.26
	%	g/kg.	%	g/kg.
Crude Protein	4.6	46.4	22.4	224.0
Estimated Lysine	.16	1.6	.78	7.8
Lignin	.7	6.8	3.3	33.0
Acid Detergent Fiber (ADF)	5.7	56.6	27.3	273.0
Neutral Detergent Fiber (NDF)	10.3	102.8	49.6	496.0
WSC (Water Sol. Carbs.)	2.3	23.0	11.1	111.1
ESC (Simple Sugars)	2.3	23.4	11.3	112.8
Starch	.3	3.1	1.5	15.0
Non Fiber Carbo. (NFC)	3.0	30.1	14.5	145.2
Crude Fat	.8	7.6	3.7	36.8
Ash	2.0	20.3	9.8	98.0
	%	g/kg.	%	g/kg.
Calcium	.11	1.13	.54	5.45
Phosphorus	.07	.75	.36	3.60
Magnesium	.04	.41	.20	1.98
Potassium	.72	7.20	3.47	34.71
Sodium	.002	.021	.010	.101
	ppm	mg/kg.	ppm	mg/kg.
Iron	26	26	126	126
Zinc	6	6	31	31
Copper	3	3	15	15
Manganese	9	9	44	44
Molybdenum	.4	.4	1.8	1.8
	As Fed		100% Dry	
RFV			127	

Fig. 3.1 A hay analysis list of findings.

The individual findings are explained in detail below:

Moisture

The optimum moisture for hay ranges from 10-15%. Hay under 10% may be brittle and dry whilst over 17% have an increased risk of moulding. Hay over 25% moisture may have severe heat damage and be a potential fire threat.

Digestible Energy (DE)

DE is the measure of digestible energy in the hay and is used to balance the energy portion of the equine diet. Most hays range from 0.34 to 0.43 Mcal/KG of DE. The amount of DE required is based upon the horse's expected workload. The average light working horse requires 9 Mcal/KG per day of DE.

The role of nutrition in the hoof

Crude protein (CP)

Crude protein (CP) is the measure of protein concentration in the hay and can range from 8-14% in grass hays to 14-17% in mixed hays. Hay containing 12% CP is considered to meet the amino acid requirements of the average horse. However, horses in heavier work, or brood mares and foals require a greater amount of CP.

Acid Detergent Fibre (ADF)

ADF is the highly indigestible plant material such as cellulose and lignin. The lower the ADF value, the more digestible the nutrients in the hay are. An ADF value of 30-35% is easily digested with values of 45% or more considered to be more appropriate for horses with lower energy needs.

Neutral Detergent Fibre (NDF)

NDF is the measurement of insoluble fibre and is classified as cell wall or structural carbohydrate. This component provides the plant with structural rigidity. NDF levels between 40-50% are from hays that are highly palatable whereas NDF levels above 65% will not be readily consumed by most horses. Both ADF and NDF levels can be used to determine the maturity of the hay, the higher the values, the more mature the hay tends to be.

Non structural carbohydrates (NSC)

Non structural carbohydrates (NSC) is an analysis of the starches and sugars in the hay. NSC is commonly estimated by adding together starch and WSC percentiles in hays and by adding starch and ethanol soluble carbohydrates (ESC) percentiles in grain feeds. Timothy and orchard grass have lower simple sugar and starch content, it is worth remembering that the colour of the hay is not relevant to the sugar and starch content. This is of significance to horses with laminitis as consuming hay containing 10-12% NSC or above not being suitable to feed, in addition suitable soaking periods may be required before feeding to those with laminitic issues.

Water soluble carbohydrates (WSC)

Water soluble carbohydrates (WSC) are carbohydrates solubilized and extracted in water. This includes monosaccharides, disaccharides and some polysaccharides (mainly fructan). This is important as fructan is a major storage carbohydrate in grass.

Ethanol soluble carbohydrates (ESC)

Ethanol Soluble Carbohydrates (ESC) are carbohydrates solubilized and extracted in 80% ethanol. This primarily includes monosaccharides (glucose and

The role of nutrition in the hoof

fructose) and disaccharides. Some analysis will refer to ESC as "sugar".

Ash

The ash content in hay forages are minerals such as calcium, phosphorus, potassium and magnesium. Another component of forage ash is the soil contamination, primarily silca. Ash content ranges from 5 to 18 percent with a good maximum value of 11 percent. High forage ash content is aggravated by both dry weather (dusty conditions) and wet soils (muddy conditions). Heavy rains have the potential to splash soil particles onto forage, especially if the forage is lodged. Factors such as rodent holes, previous flooding, and gravel roads will also contribute to higher ash values in localized field areas.

Crude Fat

Crude fat is a measure of fat content. Fat is an energy dense nutrient and contains 2.25 times the amount of energy when comparing against carbohydrates. Most hays tend to be low in fat.

Iron (Fe) and Copper (Cu)

Iron should ideally be about 4 times Copper (4 : 1 ratio) but no more than 10 times Copper. If large amounts of copper are required to achieve this ratio (more than 90mg Cu for each 2.25KG hay or 360mg for 9 KG) alternative hay should then be considered.

Zinc and Manganese should each be approximately 3 times the Copper level (Cu:Z:Mn 1:3:3).

High Molybdenum (Mo) levels are rare. Copper should be at least 6 times Mo.

Relative Feed Value (RFV)

Relative feed value is used when selecting hay and in general terms, the higher RFV reflects a higher quality hay. An average hay has a RFV of 100 although the RFV value is not used to determine the rations.

Nitrates

There are no requirements for the horse to intake nitrates according to the National Research Council (NRC) recommendations. Nitrogen often causes digestive upsets and an inability to produce B vitamins, leading to sloppy faeces and mineral imbalances.

Water analysis

Hard water contains high levels of dissolved minerals. The minerals found in some water sources include sulphur, calcium, magnesium, iron, manganese, fluoride, and sodium. Water hardness is determined by the amount of calcium and magnesium in a water sample. If you suspect your water source is hard, a water analysis can help determine if these concentrations will impact the health of the horse. Whist most water sources

The role of nutrition in the hoof

won't contain enough iron to risk iron toxicity, high levels of the mineral impact the absorption of zinc and copper.

Grass analysis

A grass analysis, similar to hay analysis will determine the minerals levels of the grazing forage. It is advisable to obtain samples of grass that is at least 2cm long, this is because it will take a long time to collect a sample and it may be heavily contaminated with soil if it is very short. The factors that affect grass nutrients include the species mix, maturity stage, stem to leaf ratio, soil profile and weather conditions.

If the pasture where your horse grazes is less than 2cm long, then you will need to rest it before you test to allow it to grow more length. The sample should only be the areas of grass the horse is eating. The areas where long grass is growing and which the horse doesn't touch, should not be sampled. This is because the analysis should only be a representative sample of what the horse is eating.

Horses were originally habituated in sparse environments with little grass and dry climates (Moore, 2013). They had to move more to intake the forage required for energy. Horses ate mono-gastric grasses and not ruminant, they evolved in low potassium and nitrogen environments. The two issues that develop with grass are lush grass and stressed over grazed grass. Both of these are too high in potassium and nitrogen with a lack of fibre present.

The potassium level of pasture is often over 2% with the ideal being around 1% with other species such as cleavers/cow parsley often measuring at 7%.

Stage of growth

Mature longer grass has lower potassium, crude protein and lower NSC levels with an increase of fibre compared to shorter grass (Fig. 3.2). The more mature and taller the grass becomes, the less palatable it becomes too, so the effects of strip grazing are beneficial here compared to track systems where horses are constantly kept on short or little grass.

Grasses that are sown with plantain and clover tend to struggle to grow well due to these up taking the ground and should be eliminated so that more suitable grazing can be developed.

The role of nutrition in the hoof

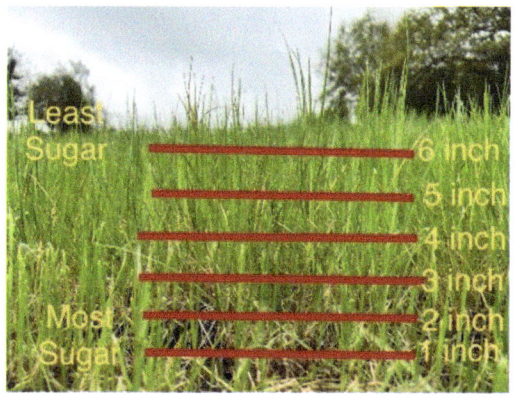

Fig. 3.2 The sugar content of grass decreases as it extends in length with short grass containing the most sugar content.

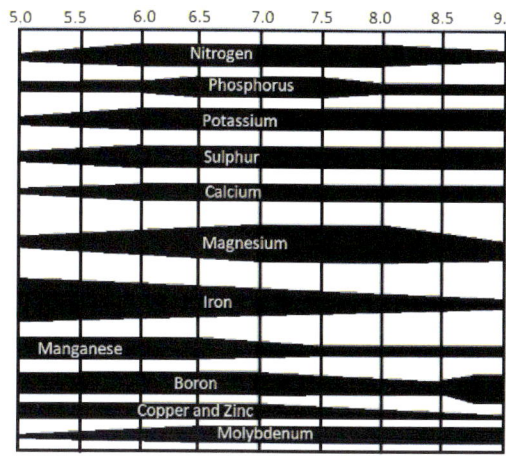

Fig. 3.3 The availability of minerals in relation to the pH content of the soil.

Soil analysis

There is a delicate balance between the balance of minerals that exist in the soil and the root in which the grass grows.

The pH content of the soil influences the availability of trace minerals and that of hoof health. The optimum pH being 6.5 that allows for a good level of antioxidants such as copper and zinc in response to a lower level of iron which is an inflammatory mineral (Fig. 3.3). There has been evidence that a higher pH results in thrush infection in the frog which can be explained by the lack of copper, zinc and manganese available.

Minerals involved in the horse's diet

There are 14 essential minerals in the horse's diet with 7 essential macrominerals and 7 essential microminerals present (Briggs, 2007). The sources for these minerals are generally found in forages and the mineral concentration is dependent on soil types, forage maturity, plant species and harvest conditions. In most cases, horses with a well balanced diet that are fed appropriately for their workload do not suffer from a mineral deficiency or excess (Fig. 3.4).

The role of nutrition in the hoof

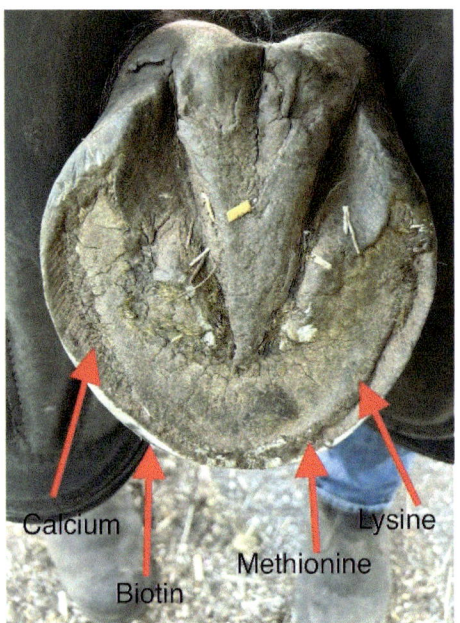

Fig. 3.4 *Where nutrient deficiencies appear in the hoof.*

Here we will explore the individual minerals, their function, appropriate levels and possible side effects from an imbalance.

Macrominerals

Calcium (Ca)

Ca is required for activation of epidermal transglutaminase enzyme. This enzyme is involved in the transformation of skin/epithelial cells into the keratinocytes that form hoof horn. Ca also helps to form crosslinks between keratin fibres. Ca deficiency has shown to be a factor in brittle hooves. Hypocalcemia has been considered a possible cause for hoof growth rings.

Phosphorus (P)

P is an important mineral for energy production and protein synthesis. P deficiency can result in skeletal abnormalities whereas an excess of P can lead to Ca absorption and therefore poor blood clotting.

(Ca) and (P) ratio

Ca and P are two macrominerals required in the diet but can vary in different types of hay. In the adult horse a Ca:P ratio should be between 3:1 to 1:1. There should never be an inverted Ca:P ratio (more Phosphorus than Calcium). Mature horses can tolerate a Ca:P ratio of up to 6:1 for a short time as long as they are receiving sufficient Phosphorus, but this should not be maintained for a long period of time (Rizzo et al. 1995). Calcium should be 1-1/2 to 2 times magnesium (1.5 to 2 : 1 ratio)

Potassium (K)

K is used for the uptake of carbohydrates, maintaining homeostasis (pH levels) and nerve function. Potassium deficiency can result in slow hoof growth and increased fatigue. Excessive K can impede the uptake of magnesium, make the horse lethargic and cause cramping of muscles.

The role of nutrition in the hoof

Sodium (Na)

Na is most often supplemented with chloride in the form of table salt and is the main electrolyte found in the horse's body. Na is used for nerve signalling, protein digestion and glucose transport.

Potassium (K) and Sodium (Na) ratio

Potassium should be around 3 times (but no more than 10 times) sodium (3:1 ratio). This can be adjusted by the addition of plain table salt; there are 11 grams of sodium in one ounce (28 grams) of table salt. You normally shouldn't have to add more than 2 ounces (56 grams) of salt.

Chloride

Chloride plays an important role in the horse by maintaining the body's acid/base balance, transmitting nerve impulses and regulating the movement of fluid in and out of cells. Chloride assists in breaking down fats in the small intestine and stomach. All horses require salt in their diet, specifically sodium chloride (table salt). It has been suggested the average 500KG horse at rest requires 25 grams of sodium chloride per day.

Sulphur

Sulphur is a non-metallic compound that is highly odoriferous with many strong smells occurring due to organosulphur compounds such as the smell of hot shoeing which is the result of burning sulphur. The concentration of Sulphur in hoof horn is due to its amino acid related role in keratin. Sulphur is the most prevalent material in the hoof making up around 4% of dry matter of hoof protein. The bioavailability of Sulphur is poor, and it is more successful to provide botanical proteins through grazing and forages (Ley et al. 1998). This is because these proteins will provide sulphur containing amino acids such as methionine and cysteine.

Whilst fresh grazing provides adequate sulphur, when the diet moves from fresh to preserved forage the addition of hay will often fail to meet the expected protein levels and therefore sulphur levels. The tensile strength of hooves has been positively associated with the level of sulphur content and the concentration of sulphur in arthritic cartilage has been shown to be one third the level of normal cartilage.

For sulphur to enter the body, it has to pass through the digestive wall where it is then incorporated into serum proteins. However, in order for this to occur it needs to be present in simple organic molecules such as Methylsulphonylmethane (MSM). Even if there is sufficient sulphur in the diet, it may not be in digestible form due to breaking down in processes such as drying of hay or maturing pastures.

The role of nutrition in the hoof

Methylsulphonylmethane (MSM)

MSM is a high quality, bioavailable organic sulphur. Sulphur plays a key role in the production of collagen, which is a component of cartilage and connective tissue. MSM is a naturally occurring molecule which is normally ingested in very small quantities, it has been historically fed in significant doses for joint supplementation (Usha & Naidu 2004). MSM is an effective natural analgesic that blocks the inflammatory process by regulating muscle nerve impulses and proceeding to active joints, where it is thought to strengthen connective tissue by maximising sulphur bonding and increasing viscosity of joint fluid (Bowe 2015).

Magnesium (Mg)

Mg is a key component in the formation of keratin, a protein that makes up the majority of a horse's hooves. Adequate levels of Mg help improve the structural integrity of the hoof wall, making it less susceptible to cracks and splits.

Mg is essential for adequate blood circulation, which is crucial for delivering oxygen and nutrients to the hoof. This increased blood flow helps maintain healthy hooves, promoting overall hoof health and growth.

Mg also has anti-inflammatory properties, which means it can help reduce inflammation in the hoof. A general guide of supplementing 1.5g per 225KG of horse's body weight per day is recommended to create an anti-inflammatory response. The type of Mg supplemented will have varying levels of magnesium present, so it is best to determine your horse's requirements before supplementation. Magnesium oxide powder is a popular choice for supplementation in horses because it is readily absorbed and highly concentrated along with it being one of the cheapest sources of magnesium when calculated daily. Mg deficiency has been linked to flat, thin soles and sub clinically laminitic hooves.

Microminerals

Zinc (Zn)

Zn is present in high concentration in hoof tissue and is considered to be critical for a variety of reasons. Zn takes the form of a finger like shape made up of zinc protein which then helps cells to multiply, maturation of a cell into a keratinocyte and for interactions between proteins, for example the production of keratin. Zinc proteins are rich in cysteine with zinc proteins becoming incorporated into keratin to help form its helical structure (Hihami, 1999).

Zn is also essential for a variety of enzymes that are required by metabolically active cells and is involved in regulating the rate of cellular division, cellular activity and cellular maturation. An example of this is zinc regulating the development of Calmodulin which binds calcium together. A deficiency of zinc can lead to slow hoof growth, thin hoof walls, weak connections of the hoof and consequently weak horn growth. Zinc deficiency is related to insulin resistance and a regional adiposity of fat developing around the body. Horses low in Zinc and Copper have been found to be more likely to develop white line disease.

When the hoof is weak at the cellular and structural level, it is more vulnerable to invasion from organisms. The copper/zinc superoxide dismutase is present in hoof tissue with its function being to prevent fat and oils from oxidizing. This oxidative damage to the fats leads to a breakdown of the protective seal on the hoof with overdrying and the glue between cells is broken down.

An excess of Zinc results in a copper deficiency because the two minerals compete for the same uptake pathways. In foals, this can result in enlarged joints (due to enlarged growth plates), angular limb deformities and shortened bones.

Copper (Cu)

Cu is considered an important co-factor for essential metabolic pathways in the horse's body. Without Cu, horses cannot utilize iron efficiently. The pigmentation of hooves is influenced by copper due to melanin synthesis. Cu plays an important role in the development of connective tissue and supports a healthy immune system. Cu can also help lower the amount of histamine in a horse's body, thereby reducing allergy symptoms. Forages contain quite low levels of copper, but it is important to maintain a correct Zinc to Copper ratio of 3:1 for the minerals to be used efficiently.

Cu is also involved in enzymes for anerobic metabolism in rapidly dividing cells and is also required for the activation of the enzyme which forms the sulphur crossbridge that hold keratin strands together. Copper or zinc deficiency has been linked to soft feet, hoof cracks, abscesses, thrush and laminitis.

Selenium (Se)

Se is often thought of in terms of toxicity to the feet, but selenium can also contribute to hoof health. Se works alongside vitamin E to provide antitoxins. Se is involved in the production of glutathione peroxidase enzyme which is an important antioxidant for protecting cells from oxidative damage. The recommended daily intake of Se for horses is between 0.1 and 0.3 mg/kg of feed. A lack of selenium in the diet causes dry, cracking and/or thin hoof walls, which become crumbly and will not hold shoes well (Fig. 3.5). Selenium toxicity occurs when horses consume 5-

The role of nutrition in the hoof

20mg of selenium per day and can lead to cracking or sloughing of the hoof wall along with lameness (Kempson, 1987). The treatment of selenium toxicity involves limiting Se intake and addressing any underlying health problems with a veterinarian.

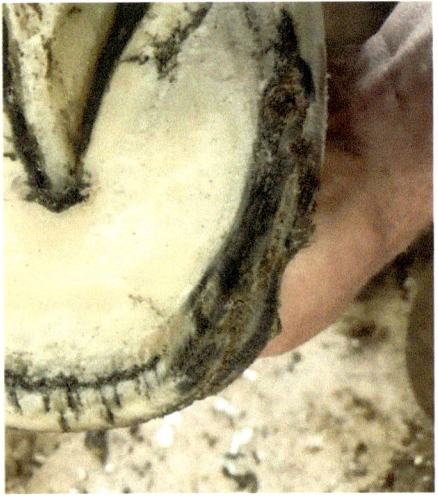

Fig. 3.5 A cracking hoof wall showing signs of selenium deficiency.

Iron (Fe)

Fe is essential for haemoglobin production which is the process of carrying oxygen around the body. Excessive Fe cancels out the absorption of Cu and Zn, even when there is a sufficient level of both available. Excessive Fe can lead to an increased risk of infection, arthritis and tendon or ligament problems. There is also a chance the glucose metabolism can be affected and potentially lead to insulin resistance. Fe is often found in high levels in grass and water sources.

Iodine (I)

As a critical trace mineral, I is essential when it comes to the production of hormones related to the thyroid – which are important to bone and brain development, and metabolism. Foods that contain I include alfalfa, algae, and kelp with a daily intake of around 3.5 mg recommended for a 500KG horse.

Manganese (Mn)

Grains typically contain low levels of Mn while the levels in forages can range from low to high. Since the bioavailability of manganese is often low in many feeds, total equine diets often need supplementation to meet the nutritional requirements.

Mn plays a larger role in developing the internal structure of the foot than in the hoof wall itself. It is required for chondroitin sulphate synthesis, which is important for joint cartilage formation, maintenance and repair. It does not appear to be stored in the body and the absorption rate is about 37%. Toxicity does not appear to be a problem but excessive Mn in the diet can interfere with phosphorus absorption. Deficiency is rarely a concern but excessive levels of calcium and phosphorus in the diet can cause a secondary Mn deficiency problem.

The role of nutrition in the hoof

Amino acids of the hoof

Amino acids are the building blocks of protein and indicate the quality of the protein sources in a feed. Horses cannot synthesize all the amino acids required for development and maintenance. Those that must be provided in the diet via feed and hay or pasture are called "essential" amino acids, while those that the horse can synthesize on their own are called "non-essential". Within this crude protein, the amino acids Methionine and Lysine are found.

Methionine

Methionine is an essential amino acid creating a building block of protein which provides support for connective tissues and has antioxidant properties. Methionine is a precursor of cysteine which forms a disulphide bond with another cysteine molecule to eventually create cystine which provides stiffness and strength to keratin. Methionine has been proven to improve the quality of hoof horn by optimising keratin (Basurto et al. 2008). Hooves that have low methionine and therefore low cysteine have weak poor quality horn growth. Methionine accounts for 1.2% of dietary crude protein intake.

Lysine

Lysine is an essential amino acid that is supplied by dietary sources. This can be referred to as a limiting amino acid due to deficiencies of lysine resulting in a limitation of protein synthesis and therefore prevent the uptake of other amino acids. The lysine requirement for horses is 4.3% of the dietary crude protein requirement.

Protein of the hoof

The hoof is made from the major structural protein keratin. Keratin is primarily made from the amino acids alanine, glycine and cysteine (which is produced from methionine). Chains of these amino acids tend to arrange in paired coils, held together by sulphur bonds. Many of these pairs together form intermediate filaments, the basic structure of keratin, and these align together to form keratin matrices, which are embedded within an intracellular cementing substance. Alanine and glycine are non essential, the horse can make these in its system, but methionine is essential and must be provided through diet. The horse can make as much alanine and glycine as it needs, but if it is not getting enough methionine through diet, it cannot make sufficient keratin, the protein building block of the hoof. The two most common keratin proteins are K42 and K124, are found in abundant supply in the hoof lamellar tissue.

Keratin

Keratin, like all proteins is a strand of amino acid units with the primary amino

The role of nutrition in the hoof

acids being alanine, glycine and cysteine (produced from methionine). Alpha keratin is the predominant keratin found in tissue from hair to hoof horn with the tubular/helix structure carried into the larger structural unit of horn tubules in the hoof wall. Beta keratin is the tougher keratin found on the outer extremity of hoof horn.

Vitamins of the hoof

Vitamin A

Vitamin A supports the production of keratin by regulating the expression of genes involved in keratin synthesis and by binding to receptors that stimulate cell division. When hay is cut, it loses 50-80% of its Vitamin A content within 24 hours and when stored in dry conditions will lose a further 7-10% every month. Vitamin A deficiency if present can lead to slow hoof growth along with brittle, cracked hoof walls.

Vitamin B

Biotin is B7 vitamin (sometimes referred to as vitamin H) that is naturally produced by microbial synthesis in the hindgut where the levels produced are sufficient for general health. A horse on a heavily forage based diet is unlikely to be deficient in B vitamins, however due to the high concentration of protein in the hoof wall such as biotin, pyridoxine, folic acid and B12 there should be consideration for this in horses with poor quality feet. Supplementation of Biotin has proven to be beneficial even if normal levels are found in the blood. It is thought that Biotin is better absorbed through the diet as opposed to natural production in the hindgut. This is due to the hindgut not being as efficient at absorbing nutrients due to the metabolism being higher up the digestive tract (Josseck et al. 1995).

Vitamin E

Vitamin E is an antioxidant that is very important in muscle structure, which is directly related to hoof movement and in the health of the reproductive system. Vitamin E is usually supplemented in the diet along with selenium, since the two work together in the metabolic process. The level of vitamin E is determined by blood testing with a normal level being considered above 2 ug/Ml (milligrams per millilitre) with a deficient level considered to be 1.5 ug/Ml or lower. There have been no reports of a toxic level of Vitamin E, but a maximum level is considered to be 10 ug/Ml.

The role of the hindgut

The hindgut makes up 60 per cent of a horse's digestive system and there are more microbial cells in the horses' hindgut than there are tissue cells in their whole body. These hindgut microbes have a significant impact on the horse and their hooves, as along with fibre fermentation they have valuable and beneficial roles throughout the body. However, just as much as they can help promote good hoof health, certain types of microbes can also negatively affect it and become the cause of disease.

Hindgut microbes include protozoa and fungi but the largest population in the hindgut are bacteria, and it is the bacteria that are predominately involved in fermentation. The hindgut bacteria responsible for fermentation can be divided in to three main functional groups: Cellulolytic (digest fibre), Amylolytic and Glycolytic (digest starch and sugar and produce lactic acid) and lactic acid utilising bacteria. Bacteria are also known to synthesise Vitamin K and essential B vitamins such as Biotin.

Certain situations such as excessive cereal starch or sugar reaching the hindgut or can result in microbial imbalances or 'dysbiosis' which can invariably lead to hindgut acidosis. Hindgut acidosis is a consequence of the rapid growth of certain types of lactic acid producing bacteria.

Making dietary changes gradually will promote good overall microbial health as sudden change is one of the major causes of microbial dysbiosis.

A diverse diet promotes a diverse microbiome so providing plenty of forage biodiversity through a mix of forages or mixed species hay and grazing will support a healthier hindgut, which in turn will support healthier hooves.

The increased lactic acid causes a drop in pH and results in a more acidic environment and can lead to inflammation of the hindgut membrane and potentially laminitis along with causing the breakdown of essential hoof structures, pain and lameness.

The diverse types of bacteria live together with other gut microbes in a balanced hindgut in a 'symbiotic' relationship within an optimal pH of around 6.5-7. Cellulolytic bacteria are the most beneficial, as these break down fibre such as acetate, butyrate and propionate into short chain fatty acids (SCFA) through the process of fermentation.

The key to achieving the happiest and healthiest hindgut microbes is by feeding plenty of ad-lib, good-quality fibre. Fibre promotes microbial equilibrium and encourages the growth of cellulolytic bacteria and research has shown that horses fed mainly fibre have a more stable microbial community. A more stable microbial community means a healthier horse and a high fibre diet helps nurture this stability.

Adding Yeasts (which are species of microscopic fungi) to the horse's diet can be a beneficial addition as they have been

The role of nutrition in the hoof

shown to stimulate cellulolytic bacteria and increase fibre digestibility. The components of yeast cells not only provide feed for beneficial hindgut bacteria but can also remove harmful bacteria from the hindgut. This helps to support a more balanced microbiome, allowing beneficial microbes to thrive, which in turn should help the horse and their hooves to thrive too.

Conclusion

Although there is a lot to take in with this chapter, the key to good hoof health is to feed a well rounded diet with appropriate levels of forage relative to the horse's expected workload and access to some biodiversity in plants that help create a diverse microbiome. An analysis of the horse's hay, grass, soil and water can help identify any deficiencies in the diet that can be made up with supplementation.

However, a good quality balancer with the right mineral ratios and dosage levels will provide the requirements for a healthy hoof as long as no individual mineral exceeds the daily limit when taking into account the digestion of other forage. Lastly, a good diet will not be successful if the hoof care provided is poor so ensure the horse is on a regular trim cycle and appropriately assessed at each appointment.

References

Basurto, R.N., Arrieta, L.S., Castrejon, H.V., Martinez, J.A.E. & Herrera, C.A.C. (2008) 'Effect of zinc methionine on the equine hoof: an evaluation by environmental scanning electron microscopy', *Veterina Mexico*, Vol 39, pp 247-253

Bowe, A. (2015) 'MSM and healthy hooves', *Horses and people*, Vol. 6, pp 53-59.

Briggs K. (2007), Equine nutrition – your guide to horse health care and management, Eclipse Press: Lexington, Kentucky.

Hihami A. (1999), Occurrence of white line disease in performance horses fed low zinc and low copper diets, *Journal of Equine Science*, Vol. 10, pp 27-39.

Josseck, H., Zenker, W. & Geyer, H. (1995) 'Hoof horn abnormalities in Lippizaner horses and the effects of dietary biotin on macroscopic aspects of hoof quality', *Equine Veterinary Journal*, Vol 26, pp 51-57

Kempson S.A. (1987), Scanning electron microscope observations of hoof horn from horses with brittle feet, *Veterinary Record*, Vol.120, No.24, pp 56-66.

Ley W.B., Scott P.R. & Dunnington E.A. (1998), Effects of season and diet on tensile strength and mineral content of the equine hoof wall, *Equine Veterinary Journal*, Suppl. 26, pp 80-92.

Moore P. (2013) 'Growing a healthy hoof with pasture as the primary forage' Proc. 2013 Bowker Lectures, Seymour, Australia.

Rizzo R., Grandolfo M. & Godeas C. (1995) 'Calcium, sulfur and zinc distribution in normal and arthritic articular equine cartilage: a synchroton radiation-induced X-ray emission (SRIXE) study' Journal Exp Zoology; pp 273-283.

Rueda-Carrillo G, Rosiles-Martínez R, Corona-Gochi L, Hernández-García A, López-Navarro G, Trigo-Tavera F. (2022) 'Comparison of the Mineral Profile of Two Types of Horse Diet, Silage and Commercial Concentrate, and Their Impacts on Hoof Tensile Strength'. *Animals*, Vol.12, No.22, pp 3204 -3222.

Usha P.R. & Naidu M.U.R. (2004) 'Randomised, double-blind, parallel, placebo-controlled study of oral glucosamine, methylsulfonylmethane and their combination in osteoarthritis' *Clinical Drug Investigation*, Vol.24, No.6, pp 90-10

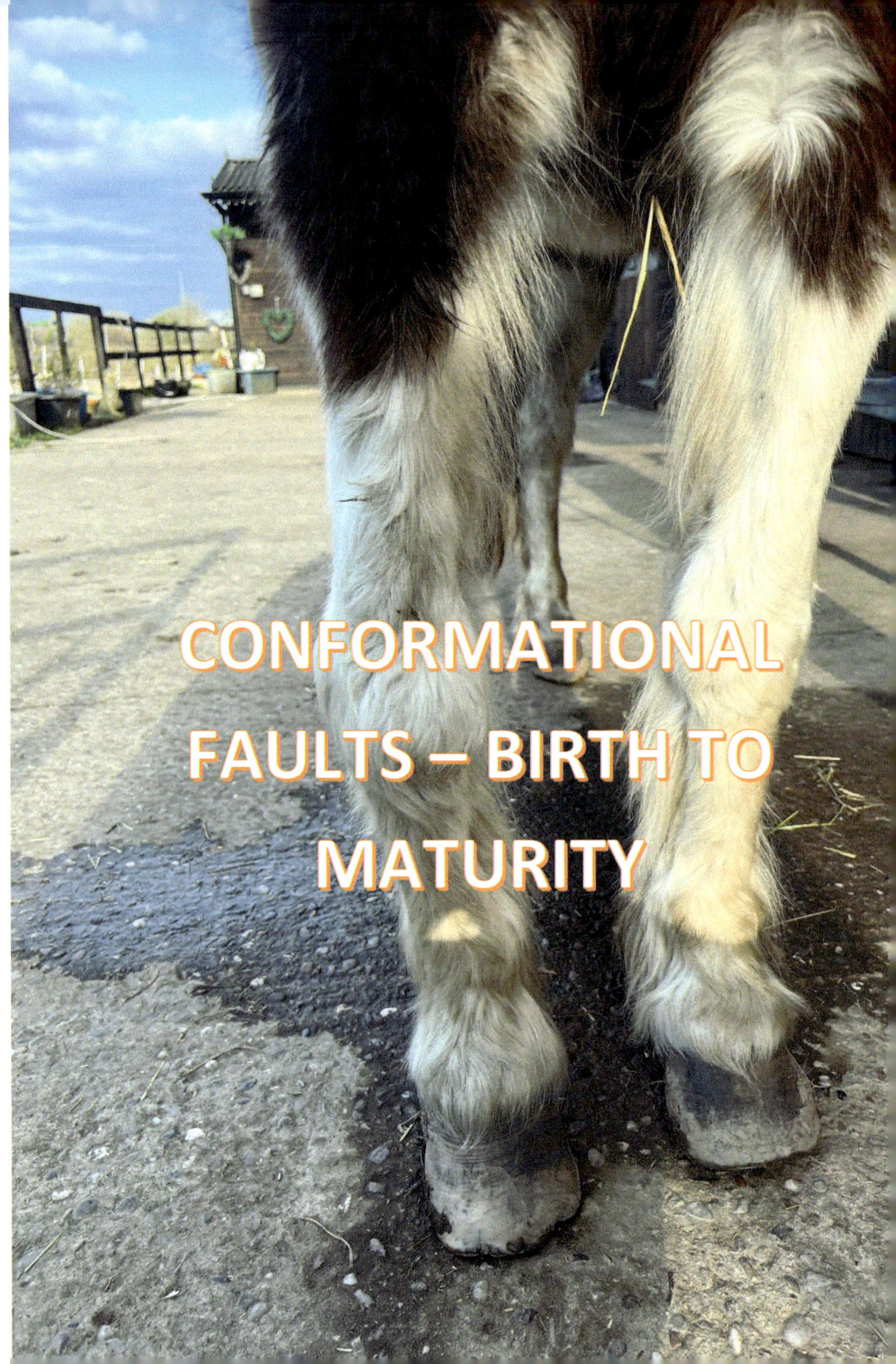

CONFORMATIONAL FAULTS – BIRTH TO MATURITY

Conformational faults – Birth to maturity

Chapter 4 - Conformational faults – Birth to maturity

Introduction

The horse's conformation is determined by the angulation of the joints of the horse, its posture and build. Poor conformation can lead to a misfunction of the feet and limbs which can then limit the horse's performance. There are some conformational faults that can be corrected in foals providing the correction is attempted before the growth plates of the bone have closed.

The growth plates help to grow bone longitudinally before closing and ossifying at their maximum length (Fig. 4.1). It is during this growth period that one side of the bone/joint can become more developed than the other side. Some severe deviations can require veterinary surgery in addition to farriery for a successful outcome. The ideal stance of a foal is slightly toe out in front because as the chest expands during maturity, the limbs and feet become straight.

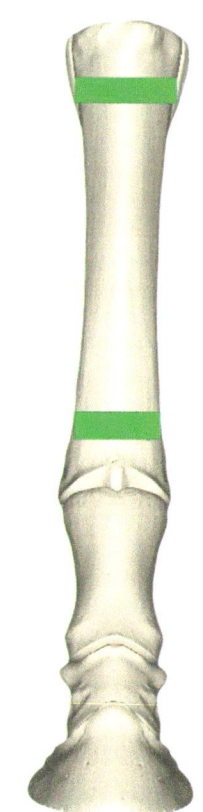

Fig. 4.1 The growth plates of the third metacarpal (green) that help to grow the bone longitudinally. *

Conformational faults – Birth to maturity

Foal deformities

In the embryo, the bones of the limb are made up of cartilage. Before birth most of the cartilage ossifies and eventually after birth the extremities ossify to form the bony epiphyses. The epiphyses are separated from the shaft (diaphysis) by a growth plate (epiphyseal cartilage). The way a bone grows depends on two factors:

- Endogenous factors – The horse's genetic makeup and hormones.
- Exogenous factors – The horse's diet or hoof trimming methods.

When the bone reaches its maximum length, the growth plates become completely ossified and the shaft (diaphysis) and epiphyses fuse completely. The bone grows in thickness via osteoblasts (bone producing cells) found in the inner cellular layer of periosteum. At the same time, the medullary cavity in the centre of the shaft is enlarged by reabsorption of bone via osteoclasts (bone absorption cells).

The growth plates of the forelimb allow for longitudinal growth and limb alignment. The thoracic (fore) limb is developed in a fairly vertical column of bones to allow the horse to sustain approximately 60% of its bodyweight.

The growth plates of the hindlimb allow limb alignment and longitudinal growth. The pelvic (hind) limb is designed to help push the horse along with approximately 40% of the horse's bodyweight being sustained on the hindlimbs.

Lower limb deformities can take place in newborn foals, and it is important to constantly assess the conformation of a foal during the first three months of birth. This is due to the closure time of the growth plates (the process of growing bone to give its length) of the bones of the lower limb. Long bones are classified by their elongated cylindrical shape and act as levers for locomotion. A full table of closure times for long bones of the forelimb are detailed below:

Forelimb (Thoracic)

Bone	Closure time (Months)
Humerus (proximal)	18-30
Humerus (Distal)	6-9
Ulna (proximal)	27-42
Ulna (distal)	2-9
Radius (proximal)	11-1
Radius (distal)	20-24
Cannon bone (Third metacarpal)	6
Long pastern bone (Proximal phalanx)	12
Short pastern bone (Middle phalanx)	8-12
Coffin bone (Distal phalanx)	Birth

Hindlimb (pelvic)

Bone	Closure time (Months)
Fibula (proximal)	40-42
Fibula (Distal)	3-8
Tibia (proximal)	36-42
Tibia (Distal)	17-24
Cannon bone (3rd metatarsal)	9-12
Proximal phalanx (Long pastern bone)	12
Middle phalanx (Short pastern bone)	8-12
Coffin bone (distal phalanx)	birth

Flexoral flaccidity

This occurs when there is a weakness to the flexor tendons and arises from the position of the foal in the womb prior to birth (Fig. 4.2). This can occur in a pair of fore or hind limbs, rarely is it observed on all four limbs. Most of the time, controlled exercise can help to strengthen the flexor tendons but occasionally farriery may be required to protect the heel bulbs and fetlock from contact with the ground (Gaughan, 2017). Trimming the hoof so the heels are migrated further back will increase the base support before applying a large palmar/plantar extension which will help the foal stand up and counteract the leverage at the toe (O'Grady, 2020). These are glued on due to the minimal amount of hoof wall available and require to be reassessed every two weeks before reshoeing every 4 weeks (Fig. 4.3 and 4.4). Any longer than this can lead to a contracture of the sole surface of the hoof from the cuff applied to the hoof wall.

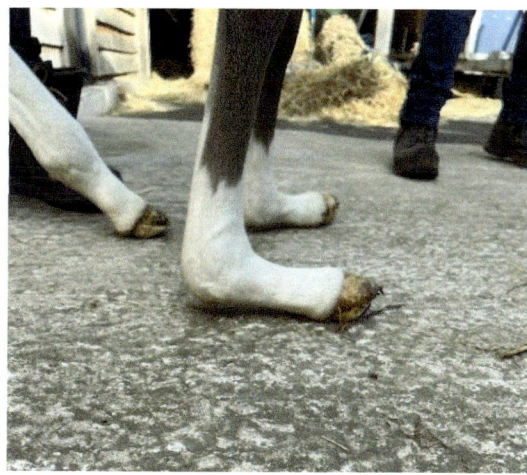

Fig. 4.2 Flaccid flexor tendons in a newborn foal. The fetlocks were contacting the ground at all times.

Conformational faults – Birth to maturity

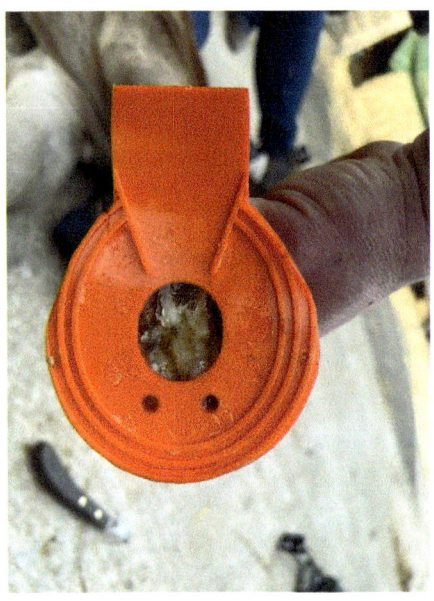

Fig. 4.3 *A pair of glue on heel extensions were applied to provide protection and a large platform base to support the weak flexor tendons.*

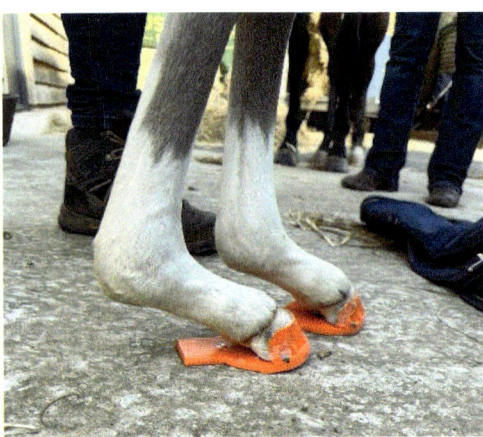

Fig. 4.4 *The foal is now much more comfortable with the shoes due to be changed in 4 weeks.*

Contracted tendons

This occurs during a rapid growth phase when the bones grow faster than the flexor tendons resulting in an upright hoof with the heels off the ground. If the case progresses, the dorsal hoof wall may pass the vertical and the foal may walk on the front of the hoof rather than the sole (Hobbs et al. 2022).

There are two reasons as to why this may occur:

- Congenital – A foal is born with flexural abnormalities which may be a result of cramped conditions in utero. Check that the limb joints are not fused or there is a concurrent curvature of the spine using radiography.
- Acquired – The most common cause which involves a rapid growth period following a setback in development. This results in the bones developing faster than the tendons (superficial or deep digital flexor tendons may be affected).

Contracted tendons are often down to overfeeding, which is then stimulating growth at a fast rate, so it is advisable to reduce the amount of feed the mare and foal are in taking during this period (Kawahisa-Piquini et al. 2023). The contraction can affect either flexor tendon with the clinal signs as follows:

Superficial digital flexor contraction – This results in the fetlock knuckling forwards whilst the hoof remains on the ground.

Deep digital flexor contraction – This results in the coffin joint becoming flexed and the foal has difficulty keeping their heel on the ground (Fig. 4.5). In some cases, they may end up walking on the dorsal wall.

If dietary changes fail to rectify to rectify the condition, it is possible to lower the heels of the hoof so that there is a very sight gap between the hoof and the ground, just small enough to fit a piece of paper in (Fig. 4.6). Then, application of a full glue on shoe with a toe extension can help to counteract the directional pull of the deep digital flexor tendon and help to restore the hoof pastern axis. This must also be reassessed every couple of weeks before removal at 4 weeks to help prevent over correction.

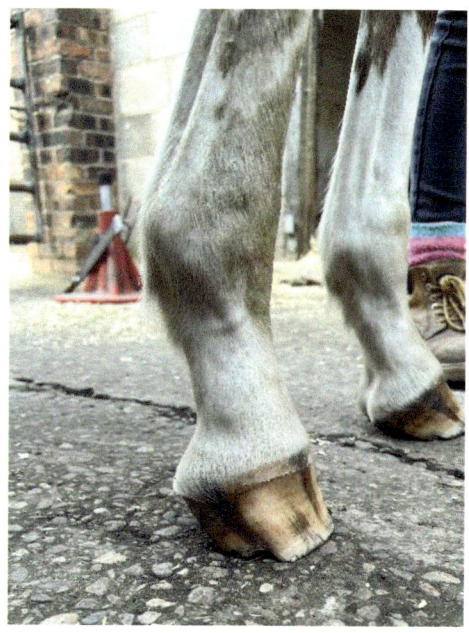

Fig. 4.5 An upright hoof as a result of a contracted flexor tendon in a foal.

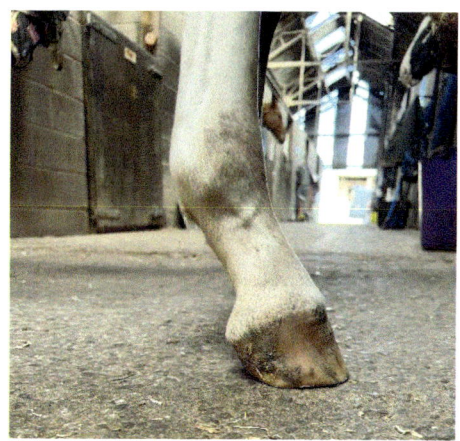

Fig. 4.6 The same hoof looking much less upright following appropriate trimming.

If there is no improvement during this period, then veterinary surgery may be required involving tenotomy of the deep digital flexor tendon.

Angular limb deformities

Angular limb deformity (ALD) refers to a lateral or medial deviation of a limb. Quite often, more than one leg is involved. The angular deformity is described by the location (joint involved) and the direction of angulation (inward or outward). ALD can occur in foals of all breeds; these are either born with the deviation (congenital) or develop the problem later (acquired) during the first year of life when rapid growth takes place.

Newborn foals have a slight 2-5 degree deformity at the carpus, however this usually straightens out by the time the growth plates close, and the horse's chest has expanded. Lower limb deviations of up to 15 degrees can usually be resolved with hoof trimming and/or the fitting of glue extensions. However, if the deviation is greater than 15 degrees then emergency surgery may be required to straighten the limb and is more successful in the early stages of life.

Most cases can be diagnosed from the clinical appearance of the limbs. However, frequent radiography of a joint can help to determine the position and development of the growth plate. The two most common surgical procedures are:

- Periosteal transection – The process of removing periosteum on "short" side of a long bone to relive tension and allow for rapid growth on the side of a joint that needs to "catch up".
- Transpyhseal bridging – Slowing down the rapid growing of one side of a growth plate by applying screws temporarily (Fig. 4.7). The screws are removed after a few weeks to prevent over correction (Wall et al. 2010).

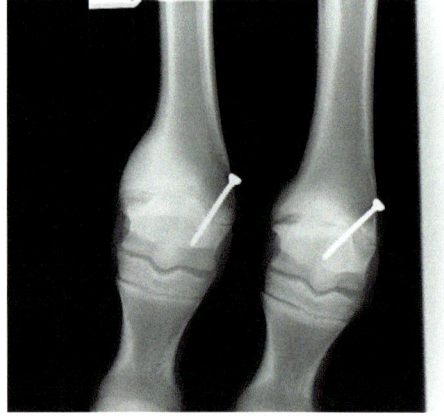

Fig. 4.7 A radiograph of a "windswept" foal that had screws applied to the overdeveloped side of a joint to allow the opposite side to catch up.

If left untreated, ALD can be a severe condition that can progress onto osteoarthritis or degenerative joint disease. The uneven loading of a limb from ALD can also lead to soft tissue injuries such as collateral ligament desmitis,

It is also important to consider the diet of the foal during the stages of recovery. Calcium/phosphorus balance should be maintained to prevent excessive phosphorus leading to phyitis and make the condition worse. The amount of concentrate feed should also be reduced to prevent the foal gaining an excessive amount of weight during the recovery phase. Be cautious to not create a thick stable bed that the foal could load their limb unevenly on.

Fetlock/Carpal Valgus

This refers to an outward angulation of the fetlock or knee. A plumline of the limb from the upper body will present straight before then deviating outwards as the horse is stood square (Fig. 4.8). As a result, the hooves will be unbalanced with a flared and high lateral side of the hoof with a crushed and contracted medial side. The initial work should focus on trimming down the lateral aspect of the hoof to provide a level footfall and monitor how the body responds over the first week.

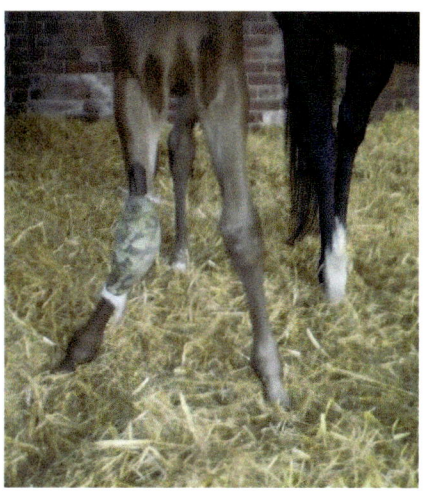

Fig. 4.8 A severe lateral angulation from the carpus (knee) in a young foal.

If suitable correction has taken place, then continue with regular trimming but if there is not significant progress made, it may be suitable to apply a medial extension to the hoof (Fig. 4.9). This is a glue on application that can take the form of a cuff shoe, or a shoe molded from hoof adhesive. It is important to create a taper of glue up the hoof wall to reduce the chances of the extension being stepped off. Reassessment should take place within 2 weeks with a maximum application time of 5 weeks.

Conformational faults – Birth to maturity

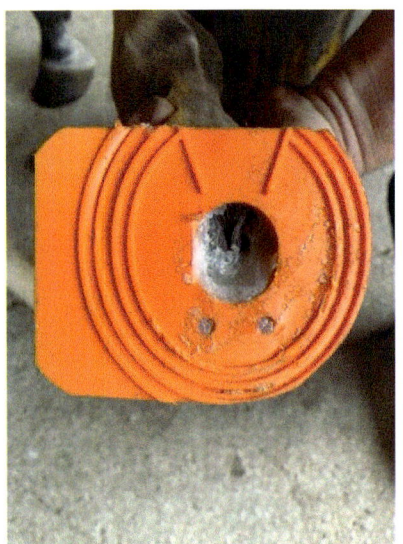

Fig. 4.9 An example of a glue on medial support foal shoe.

Some cases may also require surgery from a veterinarian in the form of transphyseal bridging to help slow down growth of one side of a bone and allow the opposite side to catch up. The screws are removed when his has happened to help prevent over correction.

Carpal/fetlock varus

Similarly, to valgus deformity this refers to an inward angulation of the fetlock or knee (Fig. 4.10). A plumline of the limb from the upper body will present straight before then deviating inwards as the horse is stood square. As a result, the hooves will become unbalanced with a flared and high medial side of the hoof with a crushed and contracted lateral side. The initial work should focus on trimming down the medial aspect of the hoof to provide a level footfall and monitor how the body responds over the first week.

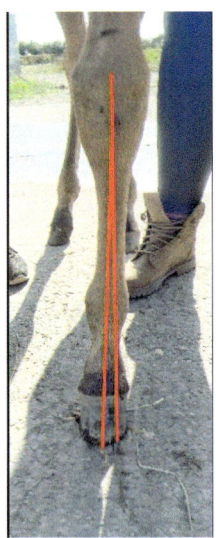

Fig. 4.10 An example of a mild case of carpal varus in a young foal. Lowering the medial aspect of the hoof with a trim should be enough to straighten the limb and allow the opposite side of the joint to catch up in development.

The same approach as lateral deviation can be applied if the limb doesn't straighten up by trimming. Careful and regular assessment is crucial for a successful outcome.

Windswept foal

This refers to a lateral deviation in one limb with a medial deviation in the opposite limb in a pair of front or hind limbs (Fig. 4.11). The same approach to the individual limbs should be taken as explained for varus and valgus deformities. As the limbs are deviating in opposite directions, any glue on shoes will have to complement this to help allow equal development (Fig. 4.12 and 4.13).

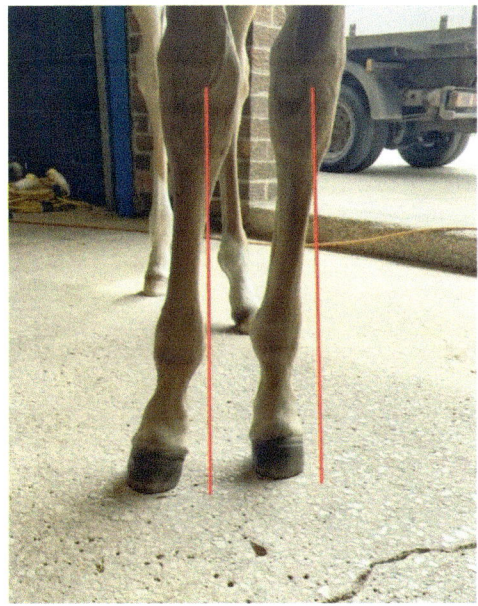

Fig. 4.11 A windswept foal with offside carpal valgus (left) and nearside carpal varus (right) lower limb deviations.

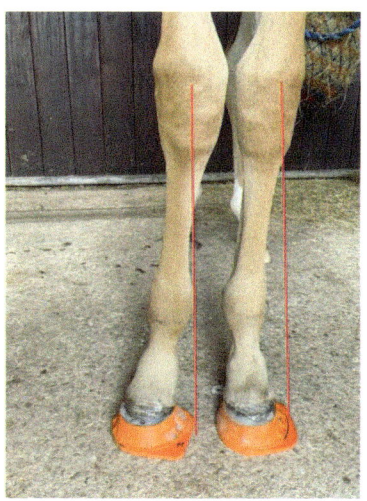

Fig. 4.12 Glue on extension shoes applied and fitted to the centre of the joint of deviation.

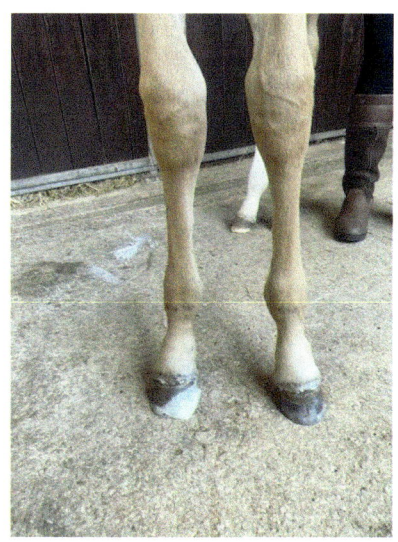

Fig. 4.13 Following successful correction over 4 weeks, only a small glue extension was required to the offside front hoof.

Conformational faults – Birth to maturity

Adult Horse Conformational Faults

Vertical axis limb rotation

This is when there is an entire rotation of the limb, most commonly in front limbs and the limb will present with either an outward or inward rotation and is often confused with a limb deviation (Fig. 4.14). Although there is no correction of this with either shoes or surgery, it is important to establish a level footfall as possible with a trim on a regular schedule. There will be no deviation of the vertical axis when viewed from the front of the horse and this is what sets it apart from the varus/valgus issues detailed above (Fig. 4.15).

This will result in either the medial or lateral aspect of the hoof becoming compromised and lacking in surface area dependant on which direction the rotation is going (Fig. 4.16).

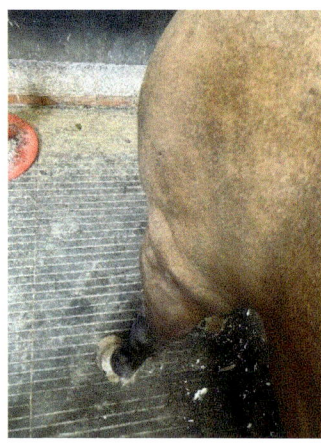

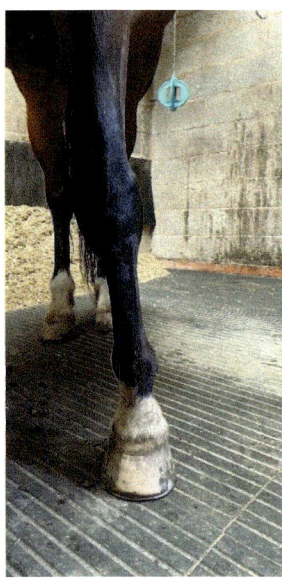

Fig. 4.15 When viewing down the rotated limb, it is easy to see why the lateral aspect of the hoof can become crushed.

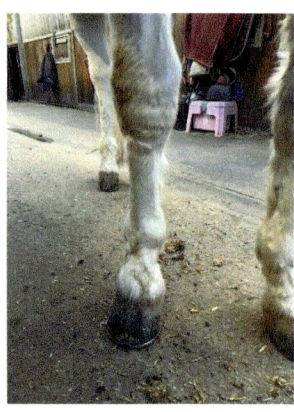

Fig. 4.14 An inward rotation of the left forelimb when viewed from the front.

Fig. 4.16 Outward vertical axis rotation resulting in a "turned out" appearance.

Conformational faults – Birth to maturity

Conformational faults leading to abnormal hooves

Horses presenting with less than ideal conformation can influence the size, shape, and structure of your horse's feet. It is worth remembering that there are very few horses with what can be described as the perfect conformation, weight, and work regime so there is likely to be a degree of tolerance from the ideal before it becomes an issue for the feet and longevity of the horse's working life.

The hoof shape is often a mirror image of the forces being applied upon it during stance and locomotion. The most common conformational faults are described below:

Broken back hoof pastern axis

The hoof pastern axis refers to a lateral (sideways) view of the lower limb. It is considered correct when a bisecting line travels from the centre of the fetlock through the pastern and hoof with no break in the straight angulation (see below). Horses with low weak heels tend to have what is known as a broken back hoof pastern axis so the bisecting line becomes angulated in a backwards or clockwise direction (Fig. 4.17).

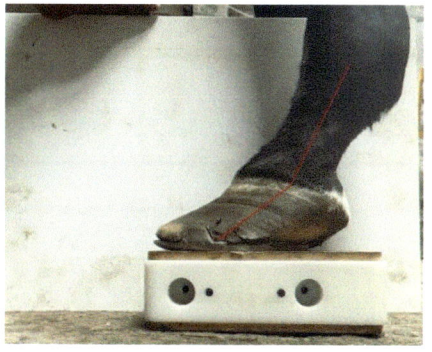

Fig. 4.17 A lateral view of a horse with collapsed heels that has then resulted in a broken back hoof pastern axis.

When horses are radiographed, this is often referred to as alignment when the fetlock, pastern and coffin joint are assessed for their position (Fig. 4.18). The radiographs will help to give the farrier an indication of the amount of sole depth available to work with and the realistic expectations of improvement with the trim alone (Fig. 4.19).

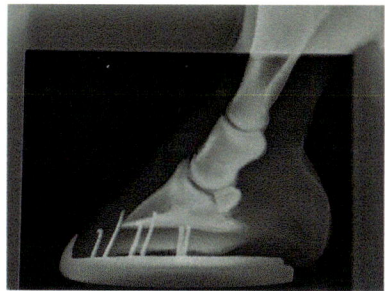

Fig. 4.18 A latero-medio projection radiograph of a horse with collapsed heels. There is a backward rotation of the pedal also known as a negative palmar angle.

Conformational faults – Birth to maturity

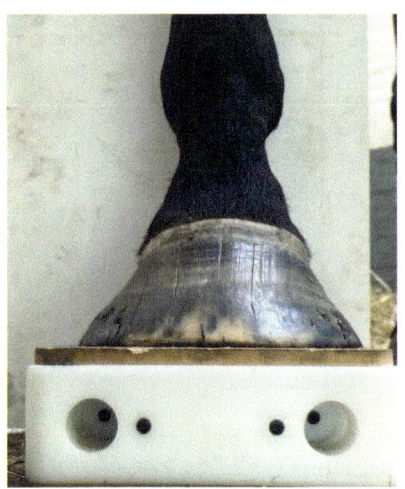

Fig. 4.19 Collapsed heels also tend to have feet that have overexpanded with significant hoof flares present.

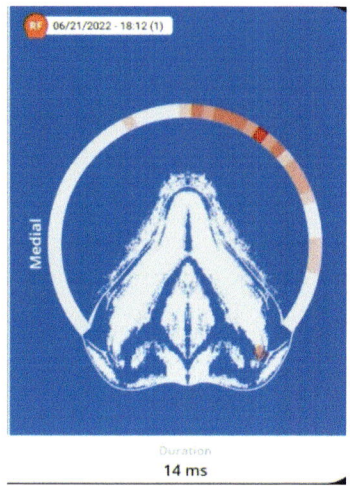

Fig. 4.20 The landing location of feet with collapsed heels tends to be at the toe.

The use of gait analysis has been shown to be advantageous when putting together a shoeing plan. Quite often, there will be a toe first landing present in horses with collapsed heels and breakover is delayed when compared to the landing times (Fig. 4.20 and 4.21).

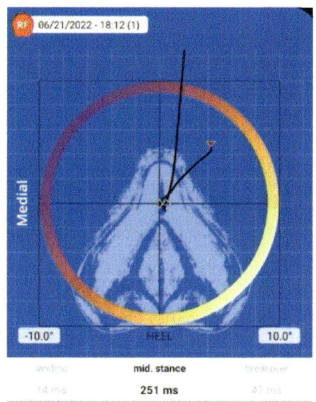

Fig. 4.21 Landing, mid stance and breakover of a horse with collapsed heels. The toe lands first before making secondary loading towards the middle of the hoof and then propelling forwards to breakover. The rear half of the hoof becomes underutilised.

Conformational faults – Birth to maturity

When considering the hoof care options available for collapsed heels, the horse's workload, environment, and soundness must be considered. There are examples of horses that have benefitted from having standard open heeled shoes removed and kept barefoot in either the short or long term (Fig. 4.22). There tends to be much more success with barefoot transitioning during wetter winter months due to the reduction of hard ground available and the limited availability of turnout pastures reducing NSC levels (sugar, starch, fructan). A track system utilising a variety of surfaces can be used to help the feet adapt to being barefoot with the long term effects of expanded heels and reduced heel migration (Fig. 4.23).

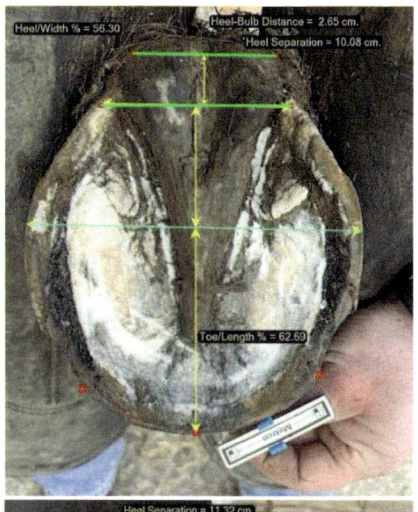

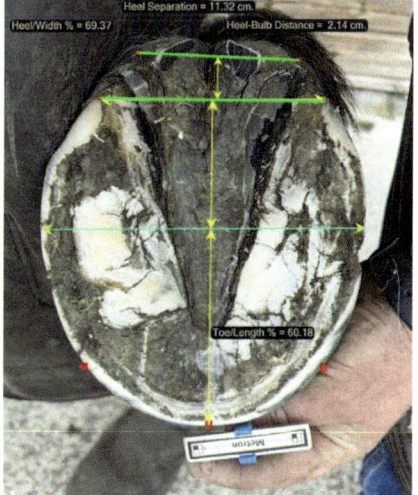

Fig. 4.22 A comparative of a horse transitioning from open heeled shoes to barefoot with collapsed heels.

Conformational faults – Birth to maturity

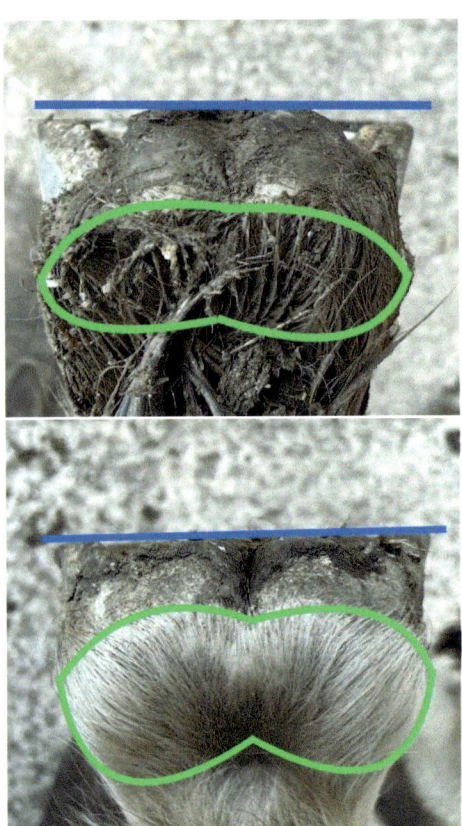

Fig. 4.23 Development of the digital cushion and heel bulbs following a transition from open heeled shoes to barefoot. Note the frog is now on the same level as the heel heights.

If the horse's workload and environment doesn't allow for them to go barefoot, shoes applied with frog support are beneficial for helping stimulate the soft tissues and developing heel growth. This can take the form of a pad or a heart bar shoe (Fig. 4.24). Ideally, radiography of the navicular area should take place first before applying steel frog support as any navicular damage usually responds negatively to being loaded up (Fig. 4.25).

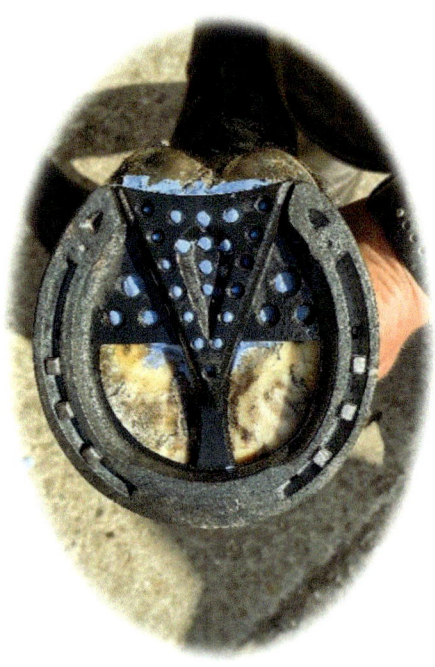

Fig. 4.24 The use of a frog support pad and soft setting impression material in the rear half of the hoof. This helps to stimulate a heel first contact and develop the soft tissues in the back of the hoof.

Conformational faults – Birth to maturity

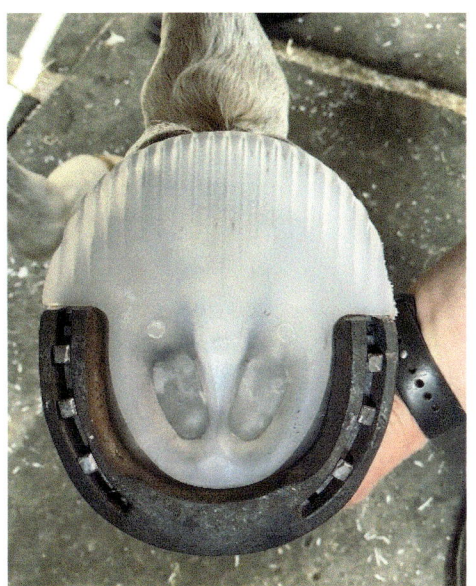

Fig. 4.25 A heel pad which also offers frog support but also allows the rear of the hoof to function like its barefoot but with the advantage of shod protection.

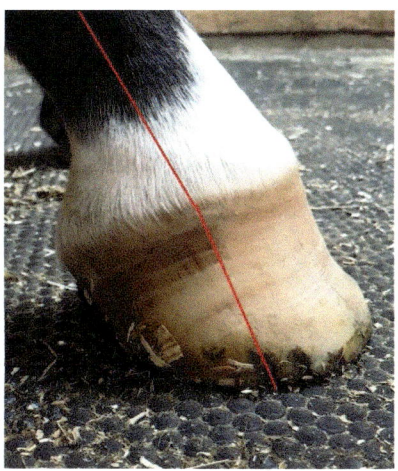

Fig. 4.26 A broken forward hoof pastern axis resulting in an upright hoof with high heels and a dish in the dorsal wall resulting from the directional pull of the deep digital flexor tendon.

Broken forward hoof pastern axis

Consequently, an upright or "club" foot is considered to have a broken forward hoof pastern axis with the bisecting line becoming angulated in a forwards or anti clockwise direction (Fig. 4.26). There will often be a short landing phase of the stride with a heel first landing that quickly transitions into the stance phase (Fig. 4.27 and 4.28).

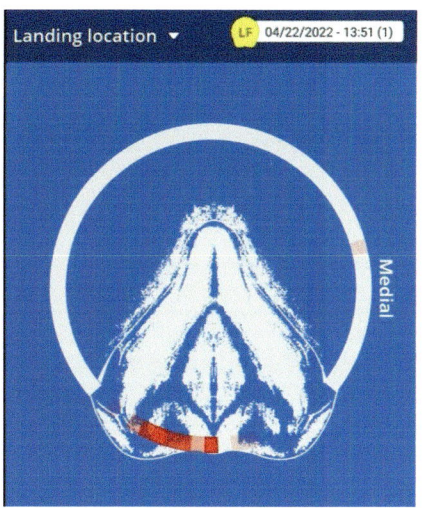

Fig. 4.27 A heavy lateral heel first contact of a horse with a broken forward hoof pastern axis.

Conformational faults – Birth to maturity

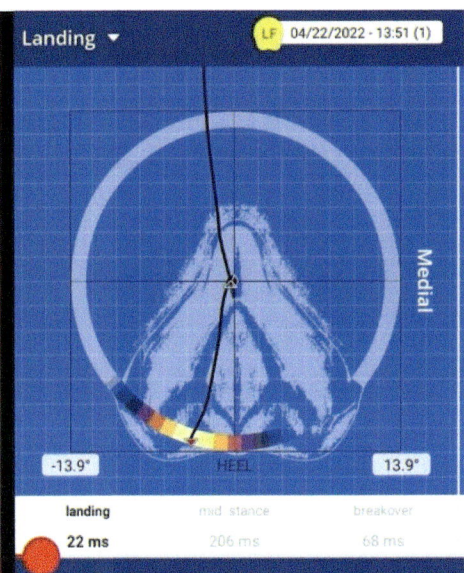

Fig. 4.28 The landing, midstance and breakover of a broken forward hoof pastern axis. The heel lands quickly before having an earlier and extended breakover phase.

Carpal/Fetlock Valgus in the mature horse

Valgus refers to a lateral deviation when viewed at the front of a horse, quite often also known as a base wide conformation. The origin of the deviation can come from either the carpus(knee) or fetlock.

The mature horse has less chance of correction, and it is a case of managing what you have and not letting the horse's stance go beyond the degree of tolerance than they have been able to cope with (Fig. 4.29). For example, a level footfall is the optimum target for any hoof care provider, and this is far more achievable with synthetic materials such as hoof pads or acrylic.

However, overcompensating the conformational fault with trimming or shoeing techniques could result in a collateral ligament injury to the coffin joint. The same could be said for horses that go too long between farriery appointments as the deviation will increase further which could potentially result in a soft tissue injury.

The recommended time frame would be 4 weeks between farriery appointments subject to the amount of hoof growth.

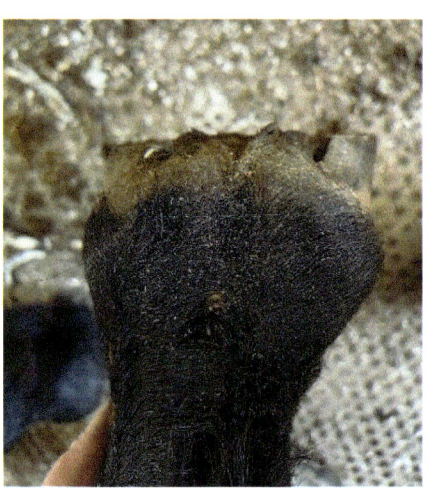

Fig. 4.29 Increased development to the lateral heel bulb on this veteran horse with fetlock valgus conformation.

Conformational faults – Birth to maturity

Carpal/Fetlock Varus in the mature horse

This is a similar deviation to valgus but in an opposite direction with a medial angulation towards the midline of the horse and is also referred to as base narrow (Fig. 4.30). Hoof trimming should focus around maintain a symmetrical base as possible with compromising the strength and integrity of the hoof. If the horse is shod, applying a symmetrical shaped shoe with the outer edges bevelled off can help reduce the effects of the limb rotation and allow the horse to lead a comfortable life.

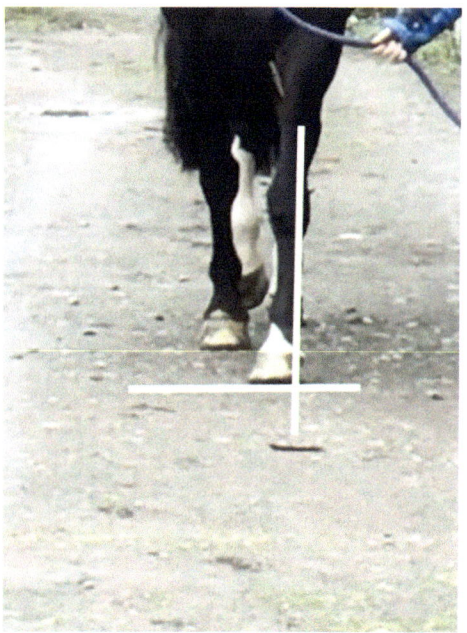

Fig. 4.30 Landing pattern of a horse with fetlock varus lower limb deviation.

Camped under behind

This refers to the stance of the hind limb being placed under the vertical axis of the cannon bone (Fig. 4.31). A horse that is camped under behind is more prone to hock, suspensory ligament and pelvic (SI joint) injuries (Clements at al. 2020). Hoof trimming should be focused on creating a straight hoof pastern axis as possible with alignment of the bony column internally.

When shod, shoes with plenty of length can help to alter and improve posture. However, the horse's turnout, workload, type and daily management must be considered first to avoid premature shoe loss.

Quite often, frog support is required due to the chances of the frog and heel bulbs prolapsing through an open heeled shoes resulting in further deterioration of the bony alignment (Fig. 4.32 and 4.33).

Conformational faults – Birth to maturity

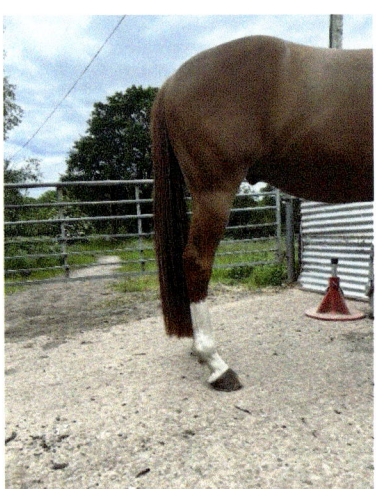

Fig. 4.31 A horse that is camped under. The suspensory ligament and gluteal muscle group will be under constant tension with this stance.

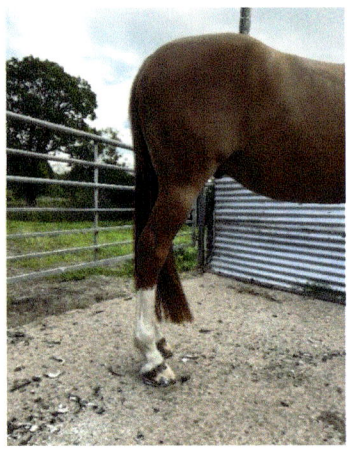

Fig. 4.32 Six weeks later following application of graduated frog support pads and hoof packing. The cannon bone is now vertical with a development of the gluteal muscle group.

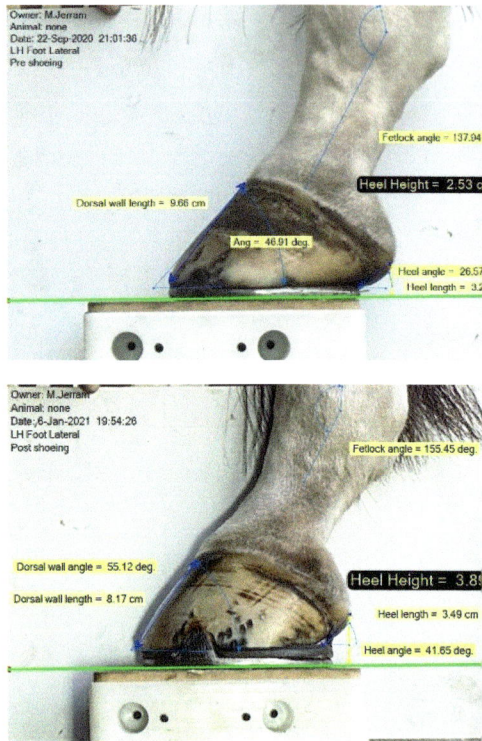

Fig. 4.33 Recovery over a period of a few months for a horse with collapsed heels in hind feet leading to a camped under posture.

Cow hocked

Cow hocked refers to a stance of the hind limb when viewed from behind the horse. The stance will involve the hocks becoming close to each other whilst the hooves point outwards more than normally. When watching the horse move, the lateral aspect of the hoof will contact the ground first and, in some cases, will screw (yaw) upon the vertical axis during weight wearing.

Quite often the lateral aspect of the hoof is contracted or worn away with the medial aspect of the hoof having more growth as it is not subject to the same ground contact forces. Trimming should focus on aiming to create a level footfall as possible and removing any medial flares to the hoof wall.

Shoe applications can include a lateral support shoe which helps to impose symmetry on an asymmetrical surface and take away some of the effects of ground friction during weight bearing (Fig. 4.34). It must be emphasised that the lateral branch should be no longer than the medial (in some cases a longer medial branch can be required). This is due to the lever effect of excessive length of a shoe causing heels to crush further.

If there is a shear or split in the frog as a result of being cow hocked, a bar shoe can also be implemented as part of the lateral support too, resulting in a reduction of the independent movement of the heels. The use of a set toe on a shoe can also help provide a fluid breakover and help to align the swing phase of the stride.

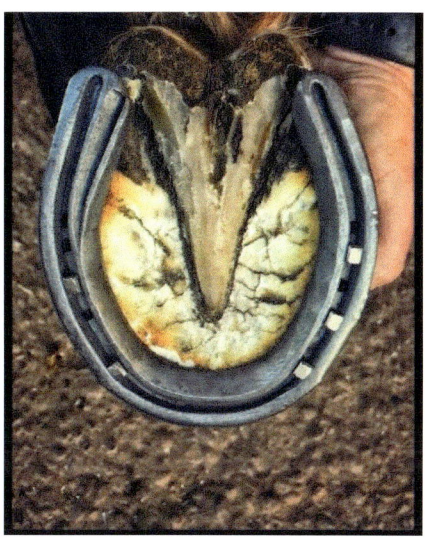

Fig. 4.34 An *example of lateral support shoe for a cow hocked horse. This imposes a symmetrical base on an asymmetrical hoof using a fuller to widen the lateral branch. Note the heels of the shoe are of the same length.*

References

Clements, P. E., Handel, I., McKane, S. A., & Coomer, R. P. (2020) 'An investigation into the association between plantar distal phalanx angle and hindlimb lameness in a UK population of horses' *Equine Veterinary Education*, Vol. *32*, pp 52-59.

Curtis, S. (1999) '*Farriery: foal to Racehorse*' RW Publications Limited: Guildford

Gaughan, E. M. (2017) 'Flexural limb deformities of the carpus and fetlock in foals' *Veterinary Clinics: Equine Practice*, Vol. *33*, No.2, pp 331-342.

Hobbs, S. J., Curtis, S., Martin, J., Sinclair, J., & Clayton, H. M. (2022) 'Hoof Matters: Developing an Athletic Thoroughbred Hoof' *Animals*, Vol. *12*, No. 22, 3119.

Kawahisa-Piquini, G., Bass, L., Pezzanite, L. M., & Moorman, V. J. (2023)' Hoof unevenness in juvenile Quarter Horses during first six months of training' *Journal of Equine Veterinary Science*, Vol. 6, 104494.

O'Grady, S. E. (2020) 'Farriery for the foal: A review part 1: Basic trimming' *Equine Veterinary Education*, Vol. *32*, No.10, pp 553-560.

Wall, R. A., Robinson, P., & Adkins, A. R. (2010) 'The use of an absorbable bone screw as a transphyseal bridge for the correction of fetlock varus deviations in six foals' *Equine Veterinary Education*, Vol. *22*, No.11, pp 571-575.

* Images adapted with kind permission from Effigos AG. Hoof Explorer.

L

STATIC AND DYNAMIC ASSESSMENT OF THE HOOF

Static and dynamic assessment of the hoof

Chapter 5 - Static and dynamic assessment of the hoof

Introduction

The principles of hoof balance and limb flight are of great debate with very few professionals agreeing on the exact same rules that apply to a well balanced and correctly moving horse. Due to the biodiversity and characteristics between breeds it is important to have an adaptable and versatile approach on how to maintain comfort with these horses. Quite often the horse's posture, workload and overall health will change during the course of their lifetime, so it is important that regular assessment takes place to detect any changes early so that they don't become precursors to pathology.

The principles described in this chapter are a result of maintaining soundness on thousands of horses over many years in the climate of the United Kingdom and act as a good baseline which can be adapted in relation to horse's conformation and workload anywhere in the world.

Careful assessment of the hoof prior to farriery intervention is vital to achieve optimum results and maintain soundness. The hoof shape and structure itself is a mirror image of the forces that are being applied upon it, simply put if there are any conformational or gait abnormalities then the hoof will deform in shape as a response to this.

Firstly, a visual inspection of the horse stood on a flat level hard surface will help to detect and record any conformational abnormalities along with any postural adaptations as a consequence of these. Then, the hoof and limb can be viewed from the front to monitor any deviations in the limb, hoof and coronary band.

Assessing medio-lateral balance

Medio-lateral is an assessment of the hoof wall bearing surface at 90 degrees to the long axis of the limb being held freely

Static and dynamic assessment of the hoof

and straight (Fig. 5.1). Lower limb deviations are usually the cause of uneven loading and therefore imbalance of the heel heights but can also be the result of excessive trimming of one side of the hoof in the well conformed horse (Fig. 5.2 and 5.3).

Due to the reciprocal apparatus of the hind limb, it is not possible to hold the limb freely and therefore the medio-lateral balance must be assessed differently to the front limb. Therefore, keeping the limb straight with the front of the cannon bone resting on your leg and viewing down from the hock is the best way to view medio-lateral balance in the hindlimb (Fig. 5.4).

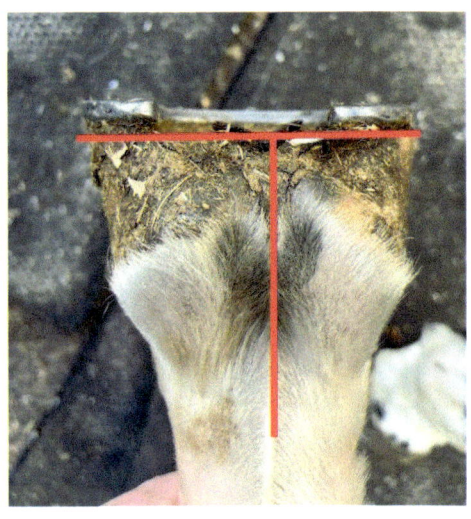

Fig. 5.2 The view that is obtained from holding the limb in that position. Note the high lateral imbalance in relation to the limb when viewed at 90 degrees.

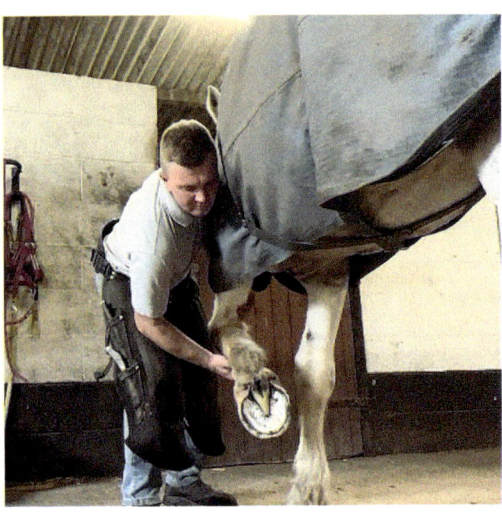

Fig. 5.1 Holding the limb freely and looking down the long axis of the limb with your head positioned over the elbow.

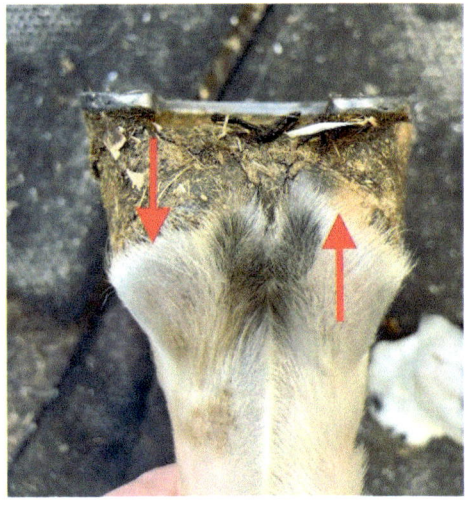

Fig. 5.3 Consequently, the heels of the hoof begin to deform into the soft tissue structures.

Static and dynamic assessment of the hoof

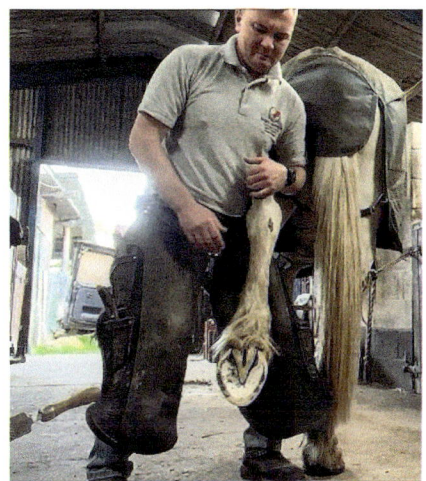

Fig. 5.4 Holding the hind limb freely to view the hoof balance down the long axis with your head positioned above the hock.

Anterior view

This view is taken from the front of the horse with the objective of determining if a vertical line can be bisected equally through the limb and hoof resulting in equal parts either side of this line (Fig. 5.5). The hoof wall angle should be the same both sides with little to no distortion along its full length. This can also help to indicate the likely action the horse takes, for example a horse with a flared and distorted lateral wall with an upright and shorter medial wall will most likely dish in their flight and make first contact with the ground on the lateral wall before then secondary medial loading and therefore crushing the medial wall as the limb loads towards the midline.

Hoof horn is compressible with their attachment by flexible laminae so if there is any abnormal pressure from incorrect alignment during the impact and stance phase, the shape of the hoof will become influenced by this.

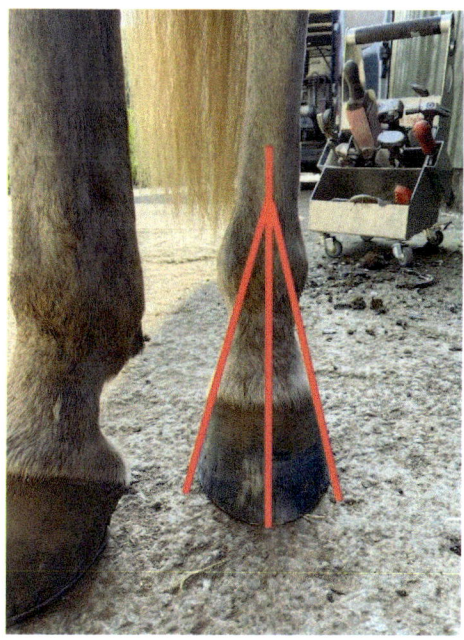

Fig. 5.5 Post trimming, there are equal proportions either side of the fetlock joint.

Recognising flares

Flares refer to a distortion in the hoof wall where there is an outward angulation of the hoof part way down rather than a straight line. This can result in separation

89

of the white line, flattening of the sole and the possibility of cracks and chips appearing at the bearing border (Fig. 5.6).

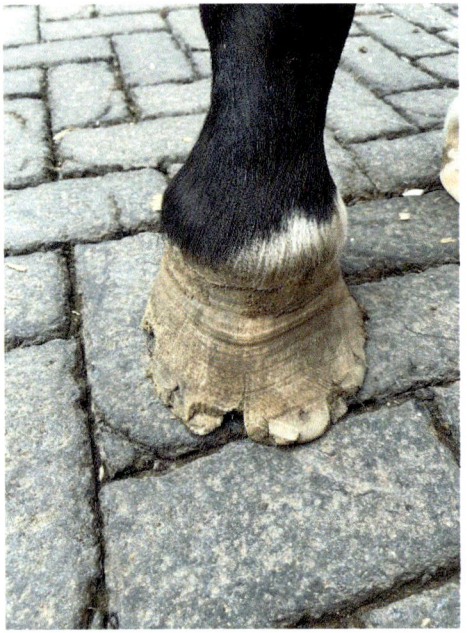

Fig. 5.6 A flared hoof the has resulted in cracks and chips at the bearing border.

Assessing dorso-palmar balance

When assessing the hoof and horse from the side at 90 degrees to the limb, it is possible to assess the dorsopalmar (DP) balance. This is achieved by determining the hoof pastern axis which involves a bisecting line from the centre of the fetlock through the centre of the hoof (Fig. 5.7). If the hoof pastern axis is correct, there will be equal portions either side but if the line falls backwards through the hoof, then this is determined to be a broken back hoof pastern axis (low weak heels). If the line falls forwards through the hoof then it is considered to be a broken forward hoof pastern axis (club foot).

When it comes to trimming the feet to achieve optimum DP balance, there is often a desire to rasp the hoof wall to sculpt the ideal hoof. Whilst some hoof wall dressing is required to remove flares, the integral strength must be preserved. The structure of the hoof doesn't become stronger by taking away material but more so from regular, careful trimming, a good diet to create structural strength and an increase of movement will stimulate the hoof development further.

If shod, the shoes applied should ideally be fitted so that the hoof stays on the shoe for the entire duration of the shoeing cycle. When it comes to determining the exact length that the shoes should extend past the heels, the expected use of the horse and conditions the horse is kept in should be considered. In an ideal world, the shoe would terminate at an ascending line with the centre of the fetlock thus providing adequate stability to the fetlock and ascending limb. However, if the horse is used for hunting or racing then this could

Static and dynamic assessment of the hoof

result in shoe loss and therefore weakening the hoof structure. On the opposite end, a horse used for dressage may require shoes to be fitted even longer than past the ascending line with the centre of the fetlock. This is due to the style of arena surface competing on and the requirement to keep the hoof from sinking in the surface, leading to tense and laboured movement.

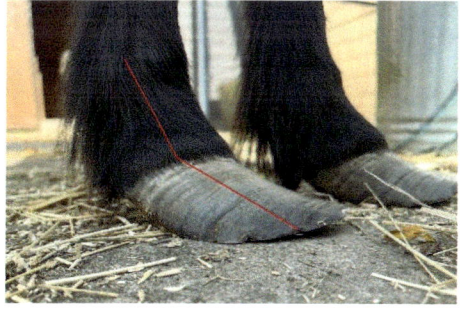

Fig. 5.7 A sideways view can help determine the hoof pastern axis and the amount of hoof required to be removed. This is an example of an overdue hoof trim.

The ideal hoof should have equal proportions either side of the midline as this indicates that is possible for the limb and hoof to load evenly and reduce the chance of injury to the supporting ligaments found at the lower limb joints (Fig. 5.8).

The contour of the coronary band should ideally follow the contour of the bearing border of the hoof which would indicate there is a lack of distortion in the hoof wall and that the hoof shape is relative to the shape of the coffin bone within the hoof (Fig. 5.9). The use of square toe shoes on front do not allow for the contour to be matched and as a result feet can become blown out and weak at the toe quarters.

There have been suggestions that the circumference of the coronary band should be 5/6ths of the circumference of the bearing border, but this should be used as a guide rather than an absolute rule due to the variation in hoof shape between breeds.

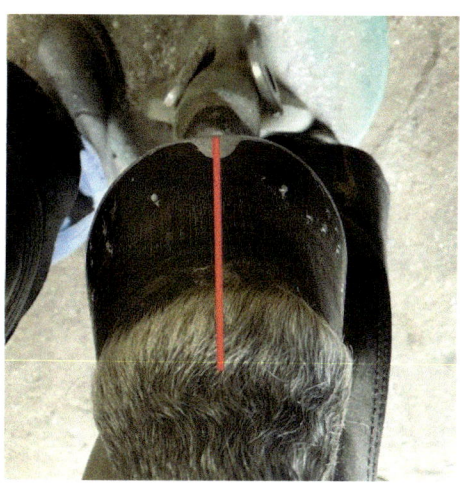

Fig. 5.8 Post shoeing, the hoof is central to the ascending limb with equal proportions either side of the midline.

Static and dynamic assessment of the hoof

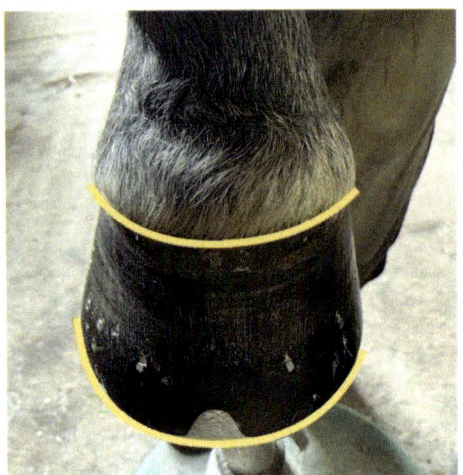

Fig. 5.9 Post shoeing, the contour of the coronary band matches the contour of the bearing border.

Shoe wear

Shoe wear is a reflection of the horse's pattern of movement, initial ground contact and breakover during the shoeing cycle. An analysis of this can help to provide a farriery plan especially if the wear pattern is abnormal.

The normal wear pattern for a front shoe is even across both branches but with an excess at the lateral toe where breakover takes place on most horses. There is often a misconception that the shoe wear should be even at the toe, but it is worth remembering the upper anatomy of the horse is rarely straight and consequently, there are minor deviations in the flight of the limb. However, if there is an excess of toe wear it can in some instances be a result of hind limb soreness resulting in the front hoof working much harder to compensate.

Hind shoes tend to wear most at the lateral toe and toe quarter due to the outward rotation of the hind limb that can result in friction with the ground during the stance phase.

External factors such as adding tungsten pins or hard face weld to the shoes can prevent wear and subsequent friction to the shoes. Behavioural characteristics such as box walking can result in excessive wear to the shoes in a short period of time (Fig. 5.10).

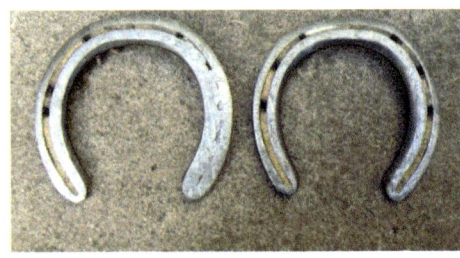

Fig. 5.10 A horse that had been box walking in one direction and has excessively worn the medial aspect of the off side front shoe.

Keeping records of the hoof

It is also now possible to keep digital records for your horse's feet and the progress they make over time by making

92

use of systems like Metron (Craig 2011). This hardware consists of a pair of blocks for the horse to stand on with indicators on the top of the block to ensure they are square to the camera on a smartphone.

Then by placing a smart phone in a mirrored cradle, accurate and repeatable photographs can be obtained. This is because of the consistent height the camera is off the ground and the distance from the hoof being a constant 90cm. A white board is used at the other side of the limb to remove background imagery. The blocks themselves have visible distanced screw heads on the side which can be used as calibration when assessing the hooves in the Metron software (Fig. 5.11).

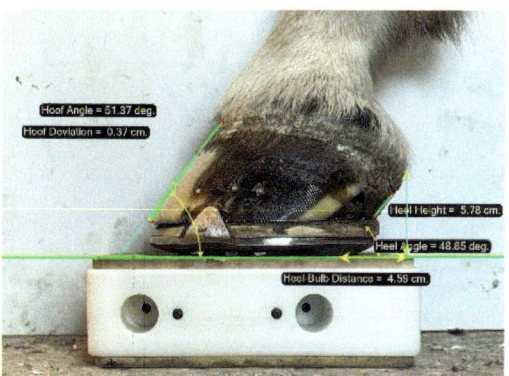

Fig. 5.11 A lateral view of a hoof with a white board placed in between the legs to remove all background. This makes the hoof easier to mark up.

Images of the sole are calibrated using a handheld distance calibration held at the same height as the hoof from the camera (Rocha et al. 2004). A white board is not required here as there tends to be less interference from background imagery with the hoof held in the air (Fig. 5.12).

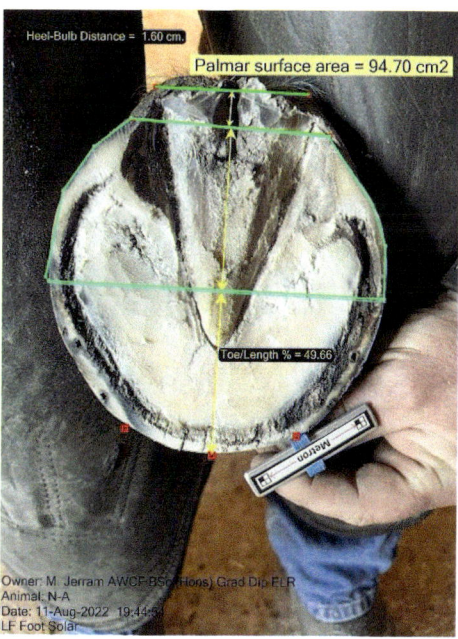

Fig. 5.12 A sole view of a hoof using a Metron badge for calibration which is placed at the same level as the hoof for accurate measurement.

A dorsal view of the limb and hoof can also be assessed for any medial or lateral deviations. It is important to bear in mind the effects of conformational defects or any vertical axis rotations that may affect the positioning of the hoof (Fig. 5.13).

Static and dynamic assessment of the hoof

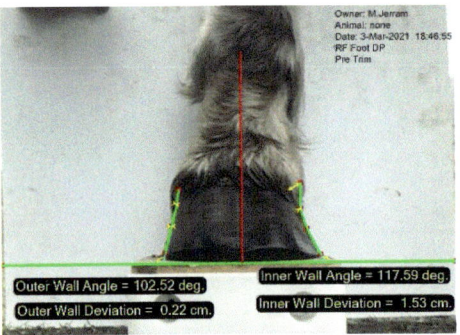

Fig. 5.13 A dorsal view of a hoof with a medial hoof wall flare.

Radiographs are also assessed using the same image capture process with known calibration allowing for a thorough investigation of the position, angulation and geometry of the bones and joints of the lower limb (Fig. 5.14 and 5.15).

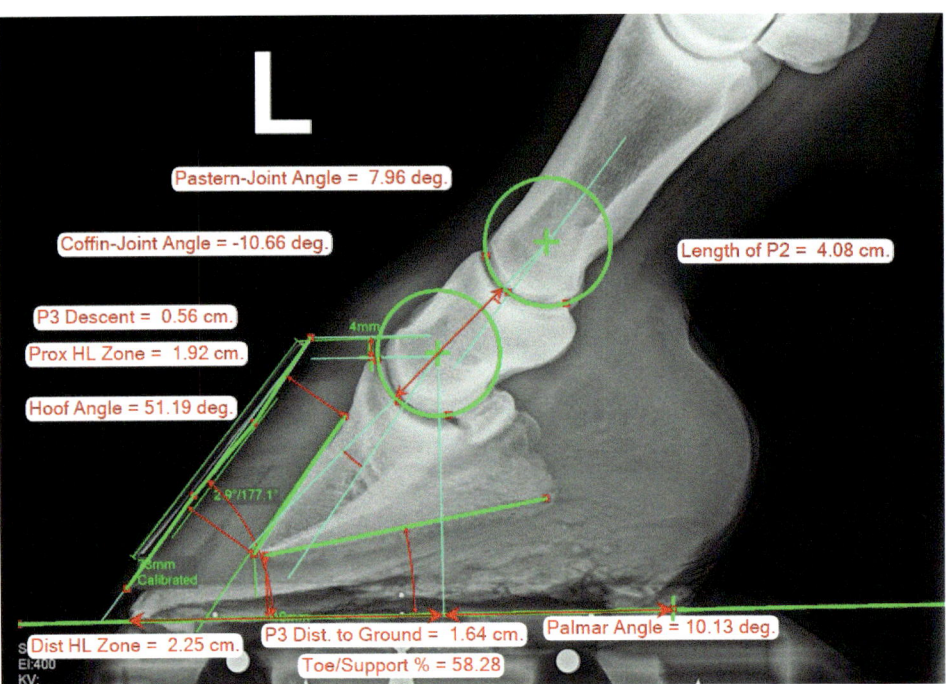

Fig. 5.14 A lateromedial projection is assessed through Metron with a wide range of parameters recorded.

Static and dynamic assessment of the hoof

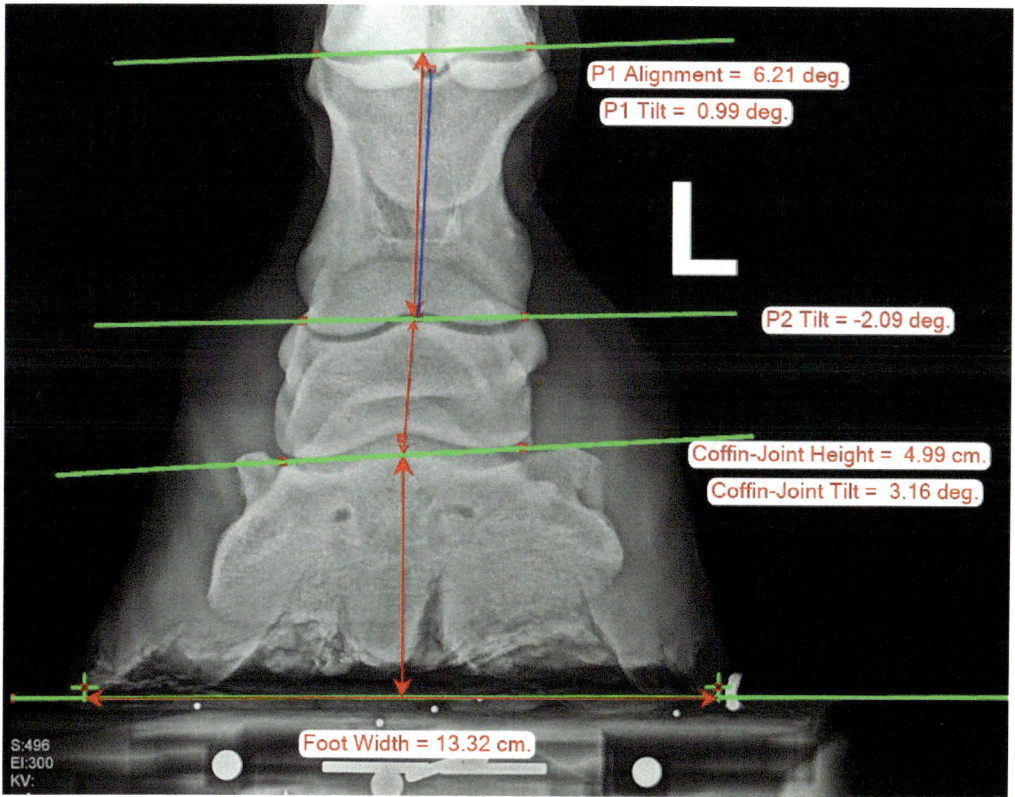

Fig. 5.15 A dorso palmaro projection processed and assessed for medio lateral balance.

As with the photography capture, ensure you have evaluated the horse's conformation and dynamic movement before drawing conclusions on the position of the joint surfaces.

Radiographs can also be stitched with a photograph of the same hoof to allow a thorough internal and external assessment of the hoof (Fig. 5.16). This is a good educational tool and puts into context the relevant findings of a radiograph (Waldern et al. 2020).

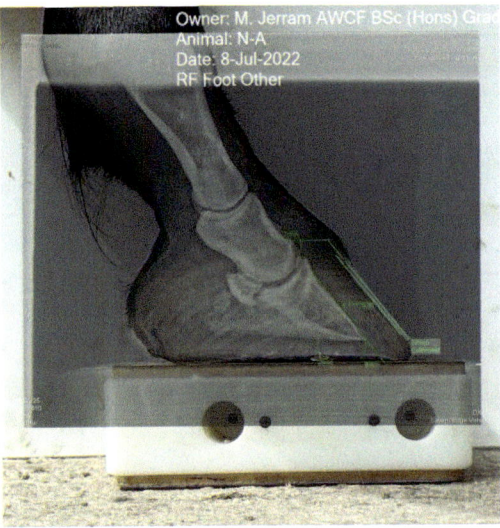

Fig. 5.16 A radiograph and photograph of the same horse merged together to give relevance to the radiography findings.

Creating a report on hoof parameters

As we have seen, the software can measure an extensive amount of parameters around the hoof once a guided markup has taken place. More recently, additional software has introduced the option of creating a detailed report of each hoof and where the hoof landmark that has been measured compares to a larger population of horses that have had the same assessment (Fig. 5.17).

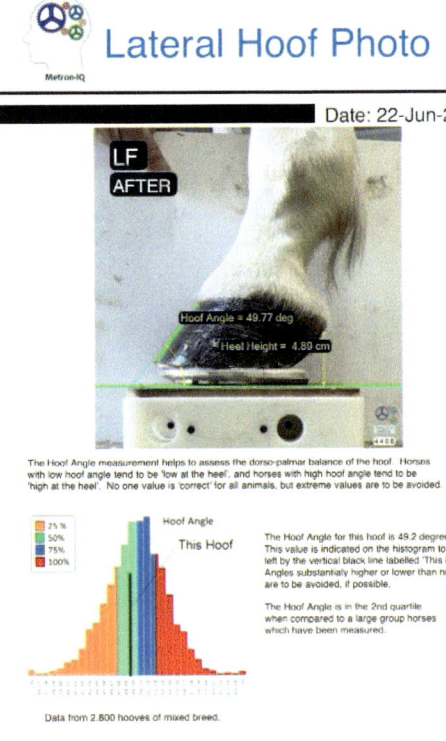

Fig. 5.17 A lateral photo of a hoof with the findings compared against 2800 other horses which is displayed in a histogram. The black line notes where this hoof lies in comparison to the findings of a large population.

Radiography can also be reported in the same way with the added advantage that the findings are compared against a

Static and dynamic assessment of the hoof

much larger population, improving the relevance of the findings (Fig. 5.18 and 5.19).

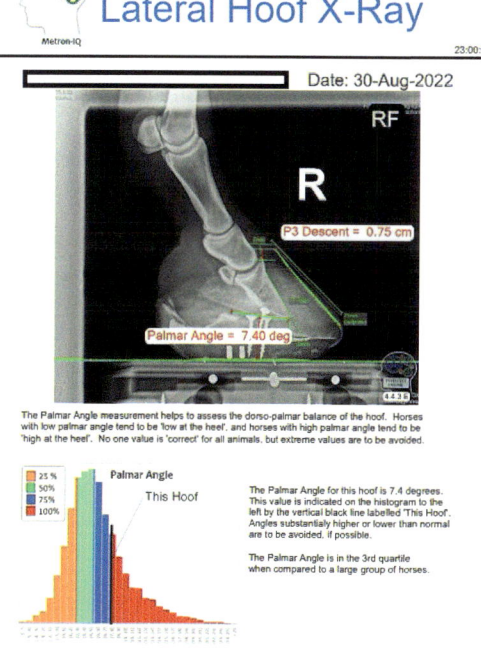

Fig. 5.18 A lateromedio projection of a laminitic horse processed into a report. Whilst no value is deemed to be "correct", extreme values are to be avoided.

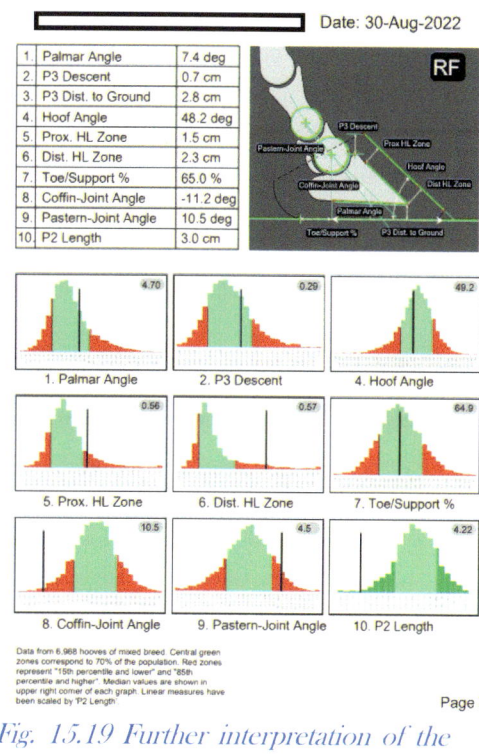

Fig. 15.19 Further interpretation of the findings against a large population of horses.

Veterinary assessment of the hoof

The use of veterinary diagnostics can be a valuable insight into the internal structures of the hoof especially in terms of alignment of the bony column and if any pathologies are present. Quite often the human eye limits what we can see in terms of dynamic movement of the horse. Where a pathology is suspected, it is best practice to investigate further using imagery so that a rehabilitation plan can be formulated. Here we describe the

Static and dynamic assessment of the hoof

various options available and their benefits.

Nerve blocks

This is also known as diagnostic analgesia when lameness is present, it is possible to locate the exact area of pain by using an injection at various site points to the limb. Once numbed, the horse can then be trotted up to monitor if lameness has been abolished, changed or altered and if that is the case, that will help to locate the area of pain. The nerve blocks are transient which then allows for further investigation with radiography.

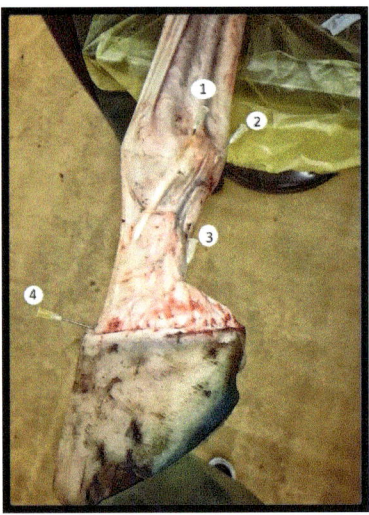

Diagnostic analgesia locations for assessment of lower limb lameness -

1. Abaxial sesamoid
2. Palmar digital
3. Navicular bursa
4. Coffin joint

Radiography

Radiography of the hoof and lower limb can be used for determining the position of the bones and their alignment. This can also help highlight any bone damage, if any arthritic changes are present or if there is a sub solear abscess present (Mullard et al. 2020).

A flat, level surface is required under cover in case of bad weather along with an area free of clutter to provide a safe working area. A gown should be worn by the handler and veterinarian to protect against radiation from image capture (Fig 5.20).

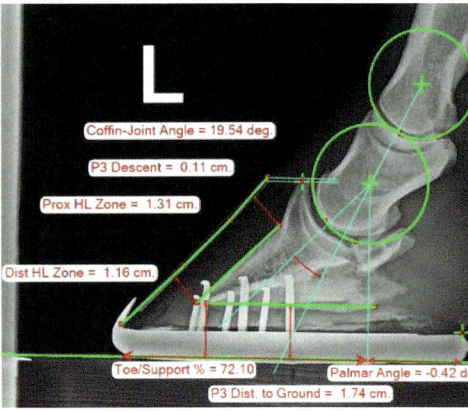

Fig. 1.5.20 A lateromedial projection that helps to assess the alignment of the lower limb joints, solar depth, angulations of joints and the hoof wall and if there is any coffin bone sinkage or rotation.

Static and dynamic assessment of the hoof

MRI

MRI stands for Magnetic Resonance Imaging and is the process of using a scan involving strong magnetic fields and radio waves to produce detailed analysis of the bone and soft tissue of the lower limb and hoof. Once radiography has taken place, it may be necessary to perform an MRI assessment of the hoof. This is because an MRI can detect any soft tissue injury to the hoof and lower limb.

Quite often, radiography will only tell half the story of the lameness with bone investigation whilst MRI will determine the other half. Shoes will have to be removed as any steel in the MRI unit will break the machinery. Horses will have to remain sedated for this process as image capture can take hours and the horse will need to stay perfectly still during this time.

Once complete, the images are sent to an analyst who will then compile a report of the key and significant findings. Quite often, MRI is the only way to distinguish the exact damaged structures in navicular syndrome (Fig. 5.21). The whole process takes around 24-48 hours to complete.

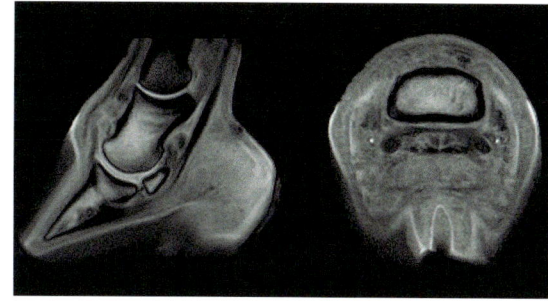

Fig. 5.21 MRI images allow for multiple views of the soft tissues of the hoof along with any bone trauma by the assessment of increased signals.

Venogram

In addition to radiography, venograms can be used for some cases of laminitis. These are performed by injecting a dye into the venous blood supply of the hoof which then highlights the active blood circulation around the internal structures of the hoof (Fig. 5.22). Radiographs are then taken within 45 seconds of administration of the contrast injection.

There tends to be reduced contrast in areas under excessive load (the rear half of the pedal bone with cases of low weak heels or the tip of the coffin bone in upright feet). Quite often there will be changes to the vascular system in cases of laminitis before changes to the position of the coffin bone. The less blood circulation present, the greater the chance of tissue dying out and becoming necrotic.

Static and dynamic assessment of the hoof

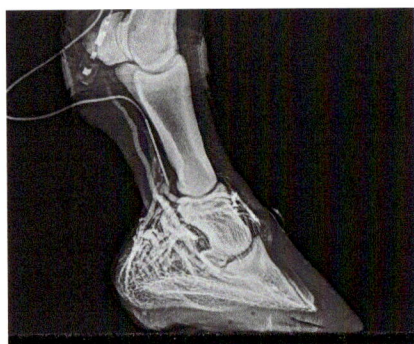

Fig. 5.22 A venogram highlighting the amount of active blood vessels in the lower limb and hoof. Cases of Laminitis have limited blood flow around the laminal interdigitation at the dorsal surface of the coffin bone.

CT Scan

Computed tomography (CT) is a cross section diagnostic modality of the lower equine limb. These cross sectional slices of imagery contain considerably more detail than conventional radiography and can be stacked together to create three dimensional images (Fig. 5.23). Additionally, these images can be reconstructed to allow the same piece of anatomy to be viewed in multiple orientations (Mathee et al. 2023). CT scans can be performed as a standing procedure giving an instant and quick analysis of the internal structures. The ability to assess bone injuries as well as soft tissue damage being possible using this diagnostic imagery. It is essential that there is no movement of the lower limb, so this procedure takes places under sedation. CT scans serve as a functional alternative to the MRI and can also be used for monitoring rehabilitation of an injury.

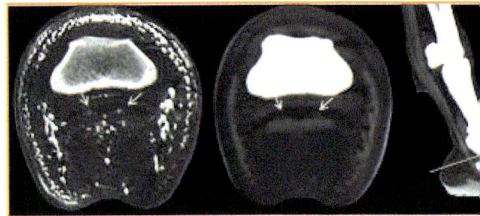

Fig. 5.23 A CT scan showing the internal structures of the hoof.

Gait analysis

An analysis of the horse's movement used to be restricted to visual inspection or by slow motion video. Whilst this still has many merits and it is good practice to train your eye to what is correct, there are now many more viable options for successful and accurate measurement of the horse's gait.

Video gait analysis can be used with reflective markers placed on external landmarks of the horse's limb before being walked and trotted up in a straight line in view of a high speed camera. The markers can then be processed through software to measure such parameters as stride length or joint flexion. The drawbacks to this are relying on accurate marker placement and the depth calibration issues of markers placed on a 3D surface area (the horse) then being measured in a 2D perspective (the high speed camera and software). However, due to some software being available for free, it can act as a useful guide particularly when training or rehabilitating a horse.

Sensor based gait analysis can provide a much more accurate and repeatable assessment of the horse (Hagen et al. 2021). These sensors can be focused on the hoof or upper limb landmarks, in some cases multiple systems can be applied to form a comprehensive investigation. These assessments can take place on firm or arena surfacing in both sound and lame horses. There are an unlimited number of strides can be assessed with a minimum level of at least 20 strides per gait. Video analysis in comparison only allows for a handful of strides, the more strides that can be assessed, the more reliable the final data will be.

The swing phase

The swing phase of the stride refers to the distance of the limb and hoof travels from leaving the ground to initial contact. Horses are designed to move in a sagittal plane as an energy saving strategy but due to conformational faults (valgus/varus deviations and vertical axis rotations) this is rarely accomplished.

Therefore, it is important to establish the significant findings of the assessment (Fig. 5.24). If the horse has a large amount of limb deviation, then they unlikely to ever move straight whereas some with well confirmed limbs showing a large swing phase deviation may be compensating for pain in the lower limb or tightness in the upper body as a secondary response (Fig.5.25).

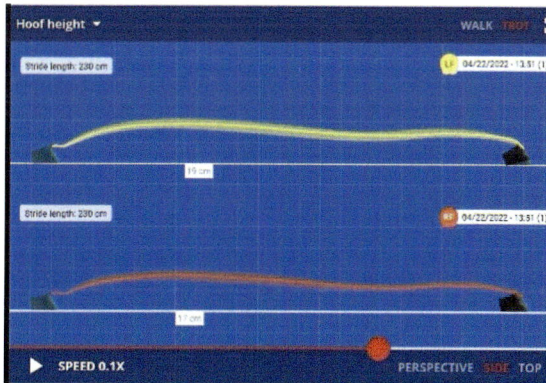

Fig. 5.24 Hoof height during the swing phase between both front feet. This is assessed using Hoofbeat gait analysis.

Static and dynamic assessment of the hoof

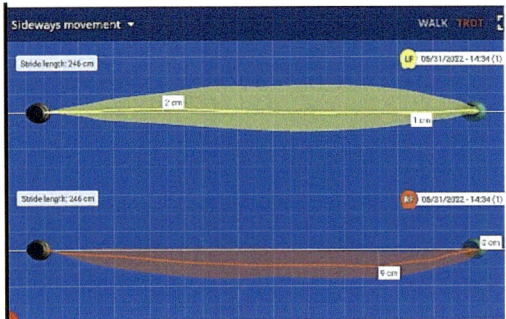

Fig. 5.25 A sideways movement assessment of a pair of front feet with the view taken above the horse. Note the large amount of abduction from the centre of mass of the right front compared to the left. The median average is 9cm on the right limb compared to 2cm on the left limb.

The landing phase

The landing phase of the stride refers to when the hoof makes initial ground contact. Immediately after ground contact, the hoof experiences rapid deceleration by vertical landing forces and horizontal braking forces that reduce its speed to zero (Fig. 5.26). The landing phase is assessed to see the initial point of contact and the duration of time it takes before entering the stance phase when the hoof is in full contact with the ground (Fig. 5.27).

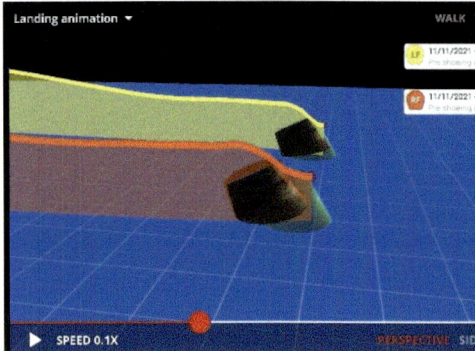

Fig. 5.26 The initial ground contact animation using gait analysis.

There are three common types of hoof landing:

- Heel first – associated with more upright feet and horses with a short toe.
- Flat – Often seen with horses with a well aligned hoof pastern axis.
- Toe first – Often seen in cases of low weak heels. The initial toe first ground contact is followed by secondary heel compression.

102

Static and dynamic assessment of the hoof

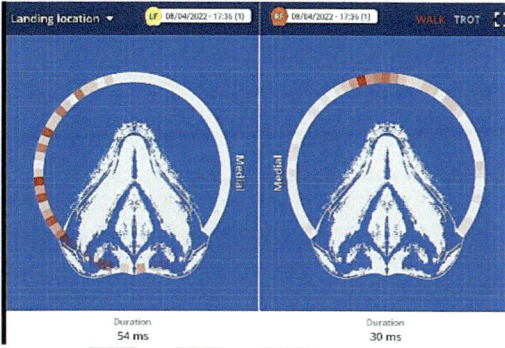

Fig. 5.27 Hoof landing location asymmetry on a pair of front feet. The left has a lateral heel first contact compared to the right with a toe first landing. Note the timing is almost half when comparing the feet.

Midstance

Midstance of the stride is when the hoof is placed completely on the ground and the weight of the horse passes over it in a cranial direction (Fig. 5.28).

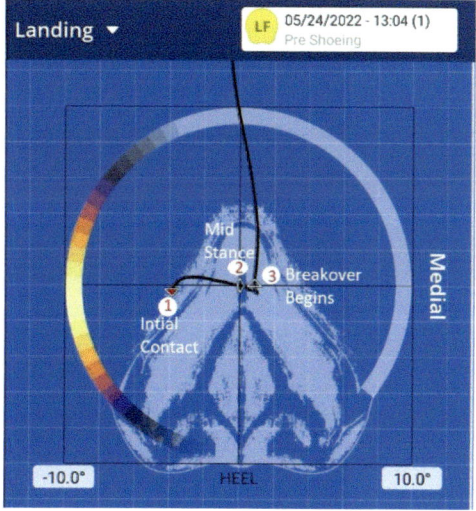

Fig. 5.28 The midstance of the hoof assessed using gait analysis. The initial contact of the hoof (1) before then rolling to midstance (2) and then the hoof starts to pitch (3) into the breakover phase of the stride.

Breakover

Breakover is the terminal part of the stance phase from heel-off to toe-off (Fig. 5.29). This is when forward propulsion of the horse brings the flexor muscles in to begin to fold the limb and the heels lift off the ground. The location of breakover is nearly always lateral toe due to the composition of the limb and the pectoral arch (Fig. 5.30). There are some horses that do breakover at the centre of toe, but it is rare to find horses that breakover medial toe unless a lower limb conformational defect is present.

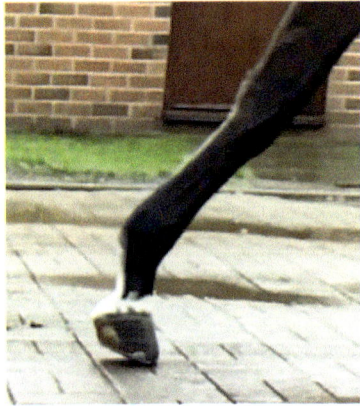

Fig. 5.29 The breakover of the stride when the toe is still in contact with the ground, but the heel is lifted off.

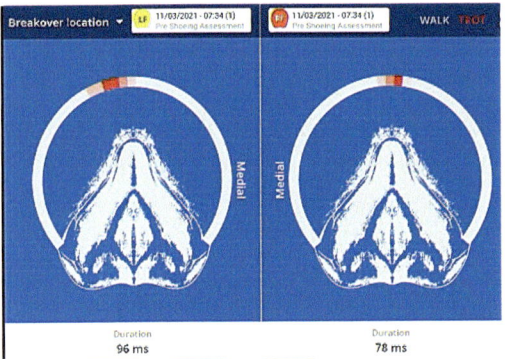

Fig. 5.30 Breakover location of a pair of front feet. Note the asymmetry in positions between the two along with a delay in the left limb breakover timing.

Stride timings

The walk gait is a 4 beat gait with large variable overlap times and no period of suspension. Even in highly trained sport horses, a regular rhythm is rarely observed so therefore the timing assessment of this gait should be approached with caution. In comparison, the trot gait is a diagonal symmetrical 2 beat gait and therefore symmetrical movement is often observed in the sound horse (Fig. 5.31).

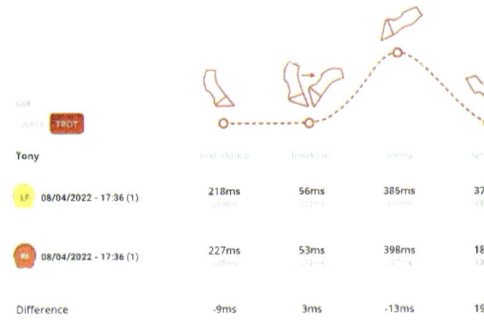

Fig. 5.31 Timings of the various characteristics of the stride. Note the difference timings add together to equal out to zero over the course of the stride.

AI Gait Analysis

Video footage of the horse can now be processed through artificial intelligence (AI) software to measure abnormalities and asymmetries of a gait (Fig. 5.32). The vertical displacement of the poll is observed when either the left or right forelimb contact or push off from the ground and compared to the opposite limb. During lameness, the lowering and lifting of the head decreases and as a consequence there is an increase of vertical movements during the stance phase on the opposite sound limb (Fig. 5.33 and 5.34).

The hindlimb vertical displacement of the pelvis is recorded from the left and right tuber coxae reference points. This is the point of the pelvis that is palpated by hand either side of the hind limbs. The lame limb will have minimal lowering and lifting of the tuber coxae compared to the opposite limb. This is known as the hip hike (Fig. 5.35).

This AI analysis can be performed on a horse trotting in a straight line or on a circle. The assessment can be performed either on a lunge or ridden with cloud based technology making it possible to assess horses remotely (Fig. 5.36). As AI develops further, the possibilities are endless for early detection and monitoring of a horse's soundness and performance (Lawin et al. 2023).

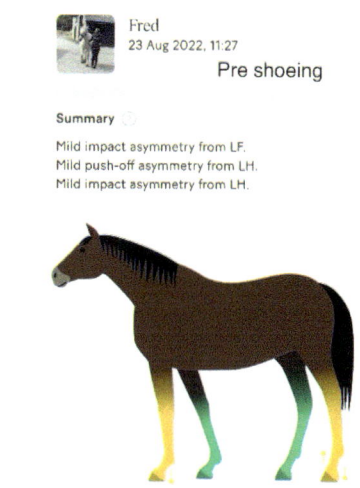

Fig. 5.32 Initial findings and summary of the AI assessment using SleipAI software.

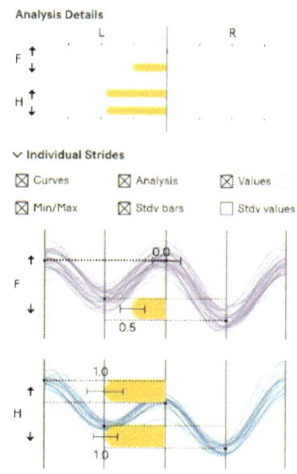

Fig. 5.33 The degree of asymmetry and vertical displacement is recorded above in the waves of the left and right limb vertical movement.

Static and dynamic assessment of the hoof

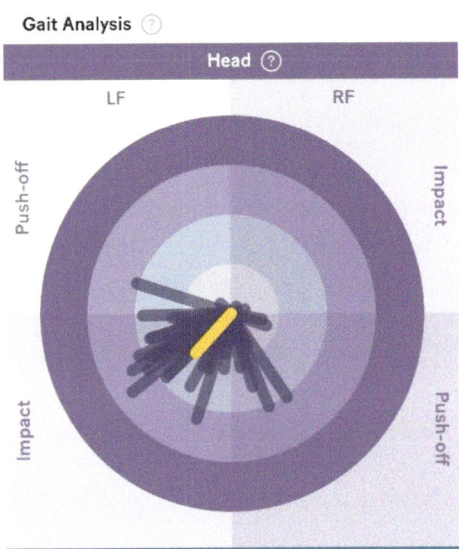

Fig. 5.34 Gait analysis assessment indicating an impact asymmetry on the left front.

Individual strides are marked on the map above in terms of vertical displacement. The shorter the length of the strikes and collected towards the centre of the map, the less asymmetry is present. The example above shows a mild impact asymmetry of the left front foot.

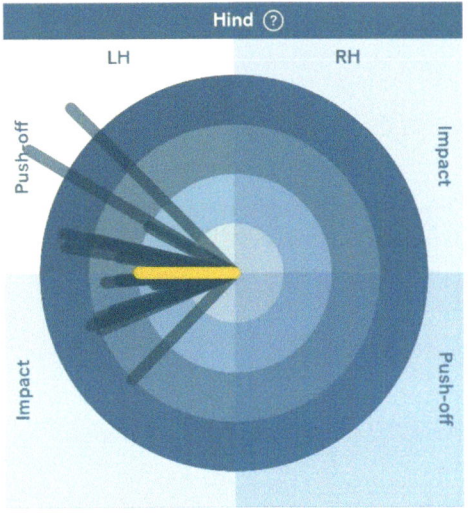

Fig. 5.35 Hindlimb assessment indicating a impact and push off asymmetry on the left hind.

The hind limb assessment is also recorded in a similar fashion with the findings showing a mild impact and push off asymmetry of the left hind.

Static and dynamic assessment of the hoof

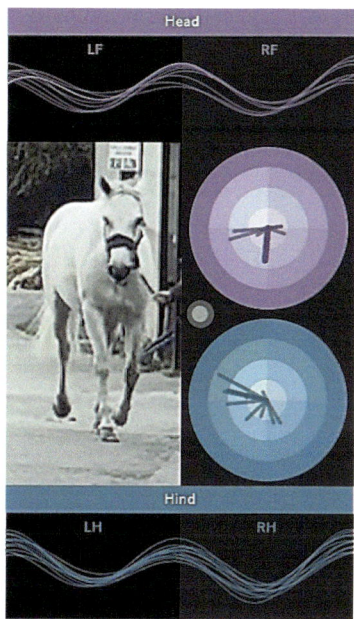

Fig. 5.36 Collection of video footage that is processed through an AI computer before the findings returned to the user.

Conclusion

This documentation helps to formulate current and future treatment plans, particularly if combined with gait analysis systems to give an extensive insight into the static and dynamic function of your horse.

References

Craig, M. (2011)' The value of measuring the hoof' *The Farriers Journal*, Vol.148, pp 6-14.

Hagen, J., Jung, F. T., Brouwer, J., & Bos, R. (2021) 'Detection of Equine Hoof Motion by Using a Hoof-Mounted Inertial Measurement Unit Sensor in Comparison to Examinations with an Optoelectronic Technique-A Pilot Study. Journal of Equine Veterinary Science' Vol. 101, pp 103-114.

Lawin, F. J., Byström, A., Roepstorff, C., Rhodin, M., Almlöf, M., Silva, M., & Hernlund, E. (2023) 'Is Markerless More or Less? Comparing a Smartphone Computer Vision Method for Equine Lameness Assessment to Multi-Camera Motion Capture' *Animals*, Vol. *13, No.3*, pp 390-434.

Mathee, N., Robert, M., Higgerty, S. M., Fosgate, G. T., Rogers, A. L., d'Ablon, X., & Carstens, A. (2023) 'Computed tomographic evaluation of the distal limb in the standing sedated horse: Technique, imaging diagnoses, feasibility, and artifacts' *Veterinary Radiology & Ultrasound*, Vol.*64, No.*2, pp 243-252.

Mullard, J., Ireland, J., & Dyson, S. (2020) 'Radiographic assessment of the ratio of the hoof wall distal phalanx distance to palmar length of the distal phalanx in 415 front feet of 279 horses' *Equine Veterinary Education*, Vol. *32*, pp 2-10.

Rocha, J. V., Lischer, C. J., Kummer, M., Hässig, M., & Auer, J. A. (2004) 'Evaluating the measuring software package Metron-PX for morphometric description of equine hoof radiographs' *Journal of Equine Veterinary Science*, Vol. 24, No.8, pp 347-354.

Waldern, N. M., Kubli, V., Dittmann, M. T., Amport, C., Krieg, C., & Weishaupt, M. A. (2020) 'Effect of shoeing conditions on hoof dimensions in Icelandic and Warmblood horses' *The Veterinary Journal*, Vol. 259, pp 105-111.

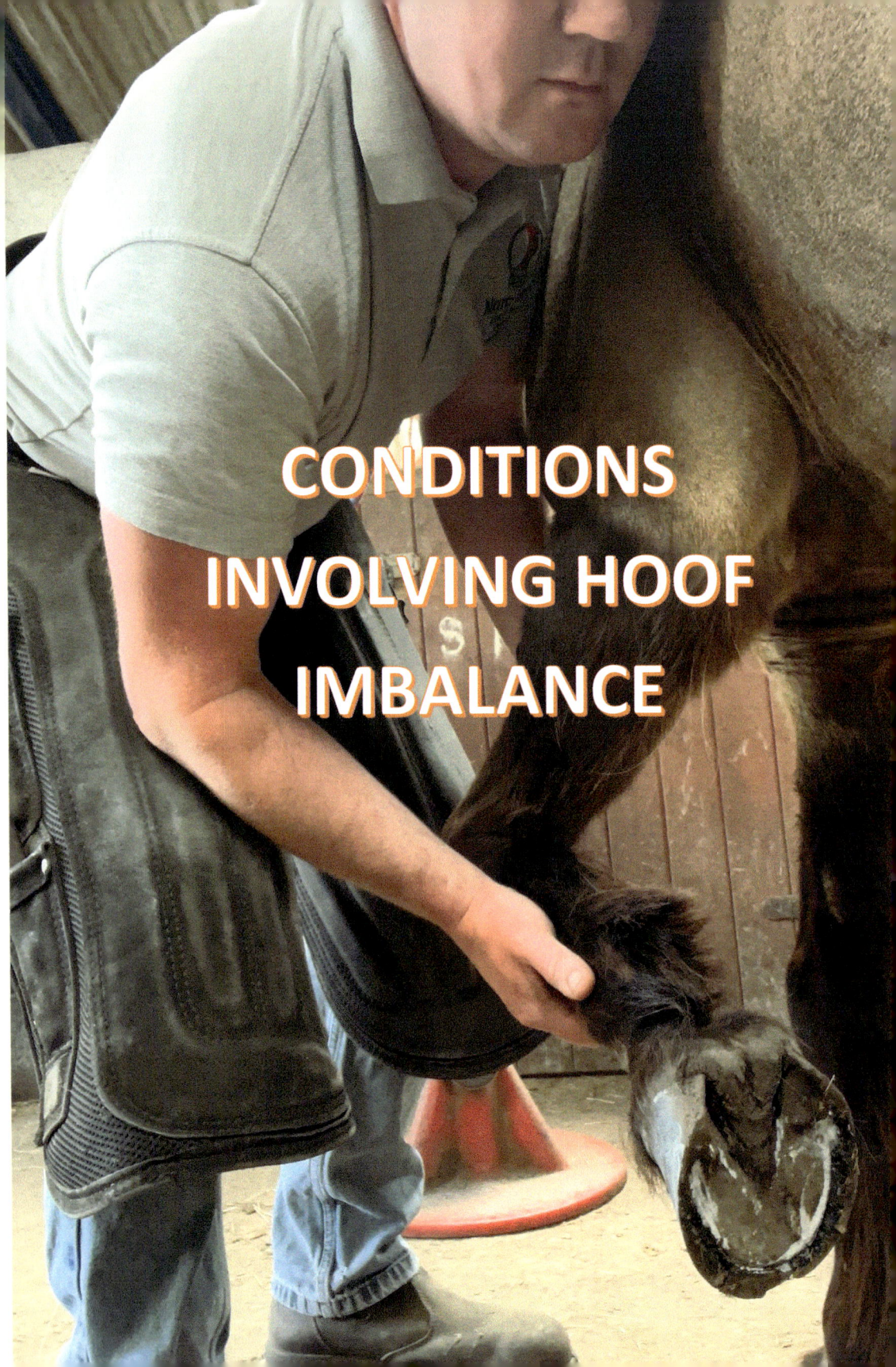

CONDITIONS INVOLVING HOOF IMBALANCE

Chapter 6 - Conditions involving hoof imbalance

Introduction

The term hoof balance refers to the ideals suggested in terms of how a hoof should geometrically measure up, move and function. Therefore, making it far more likely for the horse to perform at their optimum level and remain sound. There is little doubt that a horse with a strong, functioning, well trimmed hoof that can move and land level will avoid lameness. However, it must be considered that many hoof balance issues come from a poorly conformed horse and as a result the hoof structure deforms to the shape of the forces that are being applied upon it.

Medio/lateral imbalance

A medio/lateral imbalance happens when one side of the hoof is higher than the other resulting in an uneven footfall and possible strain to the collateral ligaments of the coffin joint. The imbalance can be the result of conformational faults (Fetlock valgus/varus, vertical axis rotation) but can also be a factor with an undetected sprung shoe or poor trimming (Fig. 6.1). There are a few ways of assessing medio/lateral balance by either sighting the heel heights as the limb is held up as close to the centre of mass as possible or by watching the horse walk up and noting the first point of contact (Oosterlinck et al. 2013).

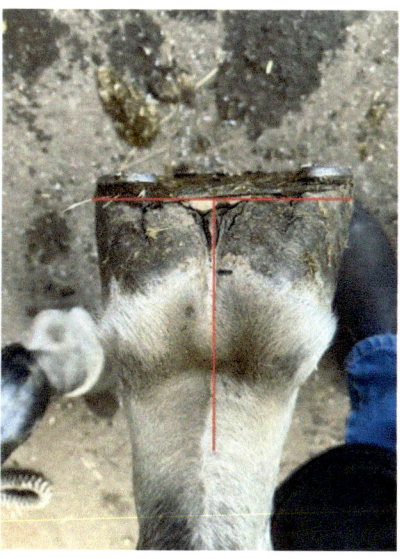

Fig. 6.1 Uneven heel heights of this hoof when viewed from the last point of deviation.

The use of radiography (dorso-palmar projection) can help to determine the joint margin spacings or the angulation of a particular joint (Fig. 6.2 and 6.3). However, it is very difficult to obtain

Conditions involving hoof imbalance

good quality radiograph with the dorso-palmar projection due to the reluctance for a horse to stand square on a block or any minor deviations/rotations will inevitably influence the findings. Slow motion video footage and gait analysis apps can also help to determine the first point of contact of any hoof (Fig. 6.4).

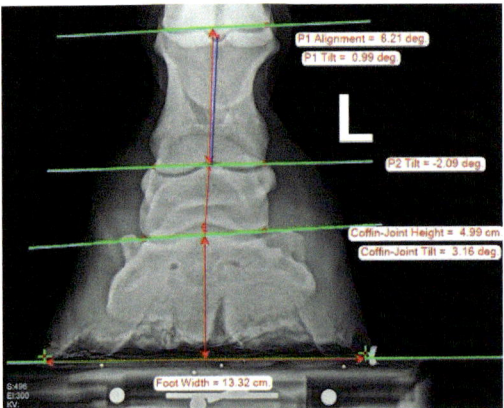

Fig. 6.2 A dorso plamar (DP) projection assessing how level the joint surfaces are to the ground surface.

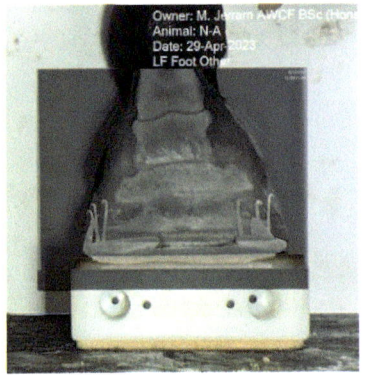

Fig. 6.3 A DP radiograph imposed on a photograph to highlight the high lateral imbalance on this hoof.

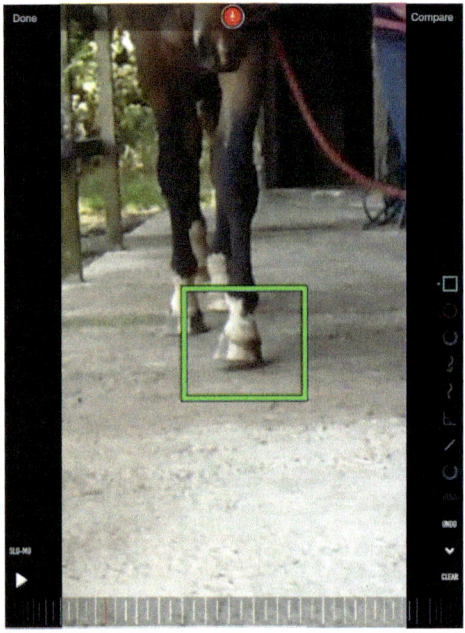

Fig. 6.4 Uneven footfall is a consequence of a hoof imbalance that could potentially lead to a soft tissue injury.

If left undetected, the hoof can deform in shape and interference injuries can take place as well as damage to the soft tissue structures. Examples of these can include corns, collateral ligament injuries, hoof wall cracks and sheared heels.

Treatment

Much of the correction of a medio-lateral balance involves trimming down the side of hoof with excess length compared to the compressed opposite side of the hoof. The horse can then be walked up to assess their progress of how level their footfall is.

Conditions involving hoof imbalance

There are cases that require additional help due to the inability to achieve a level hoof due from a lack of horn growth. The use of modern materials can create a spiral lift to the side of the hoof that is under the most pressure and help to establish a level footfall. This is enhanced further using a supportive bar shoe and/or pad to stop the independent movement of the heels (Fig. 6.5).

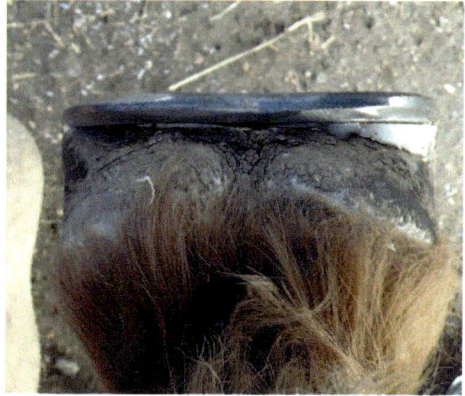

Fig. 6.5 The use of a urethane fast setting liquid to create a medial lift on this hoof with a heart bar shoe adding extra stability to the heels.

Collapsed heels

Horses with a broken back hoof pastern axis quite often have collapsed heels which is when the horn tubules bend towards the rear of the hoof resulting in a prolapsed frog and digital cushion (Fig. 6.6). This can sometimes become exaggerated in open heel shoes that are applied to horses with a broken back hoof pastern axis due to the frog and heel bulbs prolapsing downwards between the heels of the shoe.

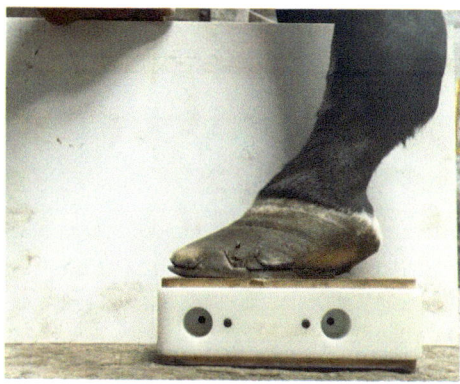

Fig. 6.6 An example of a horse with collapsed heels as a result of an overdue shoeing appointment, inappropriate farriery and the use of open heeled shoes.

Consequently, there is an increased risk of corns, navicular pain, deep digital flexor tendon injury and a reverse rotated pedal bone (Fig. 6.7). Performance related issues such as tripping or stumbling are more likely too due to the toe first landing of these feet.

Treatment

Treatment of collapsed heels most commonly involves engagement of the frog to help stimulate tissue in the rear third of the hoof.

Conditions involving hoof imbalance

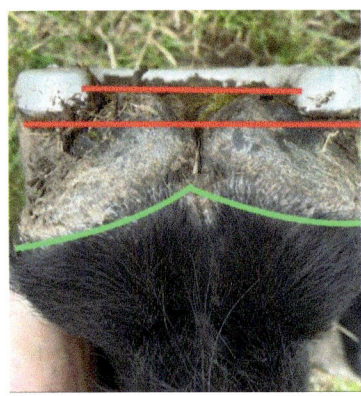

Fig. 6.7 Frog and heel bulbs prolapsing through this graduated shoe resulting in a loss of function to the structures in the rear of the hoof.

Low heeled feet are often also overexpanded in their shape, meaning they become much wider than they are long (Fig. 6.8).

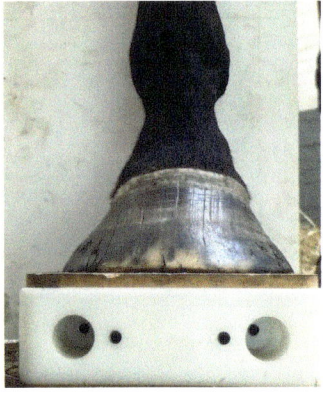

Fig. 6.8 Horses with collapsed heels often have excessive hoof wall flares.

It is advisable to obtain radiographs of the feet to determine the position of the pedal bone and whether any navicular damage is present (Fig. 6.9). The latter being critical to avoid any heel pain from any corrective application or trim (Floyd, 2010).

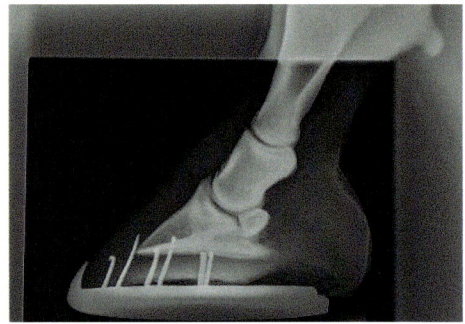

Fig. 6.8 A radiograph of a horse with collapsed heels showing a reverse rotation of the coffin bone with the rear of the bone closer to the ground surface compared to the front of the bone.

If shoes are applied, it is advisable to fit them with the heel branches at an ascending line with the centre of the fetlock which then in turn bisects the shoulder joint equally, offering full limb stability. The breakover of the shoe should be heavily bevelled and fitted as close to the leading edge of the pedal bone as possible. This will help to provide biomechanical efficiency around the coffin joint and reduce the chances of tripping. The frog support applied can vary dependant on the type of hoof, its strength, expected workload and their environment (Hunt, 2012). A frog

114

support pad is the lightest style of application that can engage the whole sole surface rather than the outer perimeter of a standard shoe (Fig. 6.10).

and strain the suspensory apparatus. Therefore, any graduation applied to the hoof should be applied with a full frog support to prevent prolapse of the frog and heel bulbs.

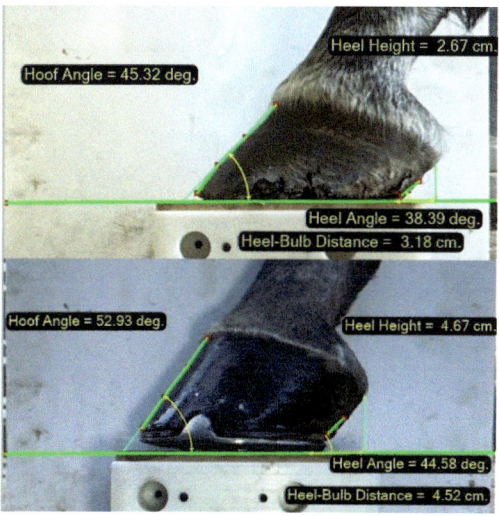

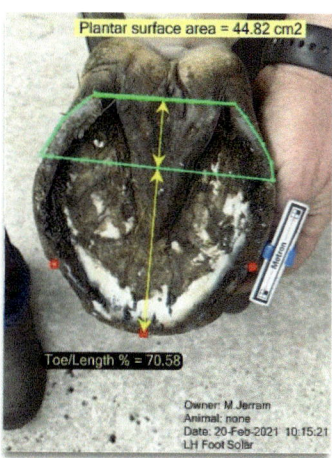

Fig. 6.10 Progress over time on a horse with collapsed heels using frog support pads and impression material.

Wedges and collapsed heels

The use of wedged shoes with either a specialised shoe or plastic wedges is often a hotly debated topic with many conflicted views on what is suitable for long term recovery. The theory being that a good hoof pastern axis can be achieved instantly (Fig. 6.11).

It is the experience of the author that the use of wedged shoes without frog support can result in heels collapsing further along with increased deterioration of the sensitive structures at the rear of the hoof

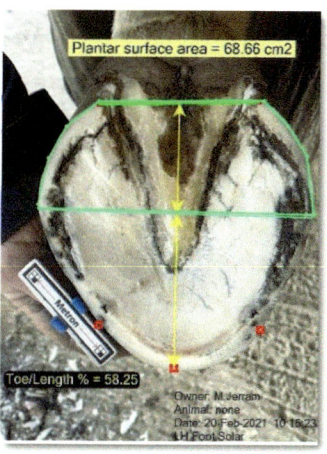

Fig. 6.11 Progress over time of a hind hoof with collapsed heels, the surface area increases with a reduced forward migration of the heels from the heel bulbs.

Conditions involving hoof imbalance

Due to access being restricted to the sole, it is advisable to apply a layer of anti fungal clay to the whole sole to keep it free from bacteria before applying a soft setting impression material that moulds to the shape of the frog and sole under the hoof pad (Fig. 6.12).

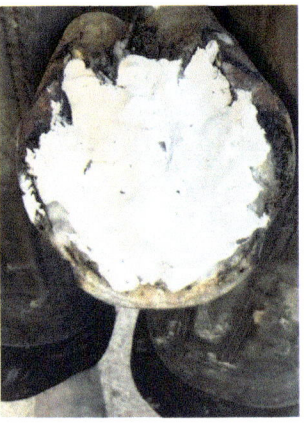

Fig. 6.12 Anti-fungal clay applied to the sole and frog to maintain good health throughout the shoeing cycle.

It can be noted some weeks later when the package is removed how clean the sole is by taking these steps and preventing any side effects from corrective applications.

Club feet

As an opposite to collapsed heels, club feet have an excess of heel at the rear third of the hoof and a more upright hoof wall angle. The frog will be vaulted with a lack of engagement with the ground and a slight dish to the hoof wall at the toe will be present (Fig. 6.13). This is due to the contracture of the deep digital flexor tendon that is attached to the semi lunar line at the base of the pedal bone.

Club feet can occur in front and hind feet but is much more common in front feet. The development of a club foot is from an acquired flexoral deformity, often from a young age that has not been assessed or corrected (Caldwell, 2017). The gait characteristics of a club foot include a stilted gait with increased retraction and limited extension compared to a well aligned hoof. As a result, shoe loss is much more common in club feet, so it is important to ensure the hoof is well protected when turned out or in work.

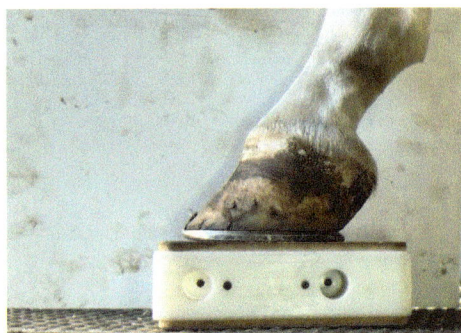

Fig. 6.13 A club foot with increased heel development and a dished hoof wall.

There is also a common association with an outward rotation of the limb and a high lateral hoof imbalance. This in turn leads to an increase in muscle development at the shoulder compared

Conditions involving hoof imbalance

to the opposite limb making it more difficult for saddle fitting.

Club feet are categorised on a grade system of 1-4 which is detailed below:

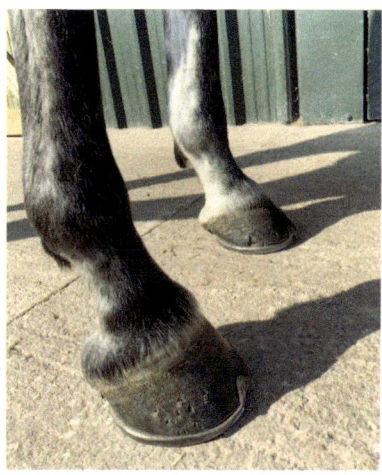

Grade 1 – There will be a 3-5° dorsal hoof wall difference between the front feet with the club foot having the more upright hoof.

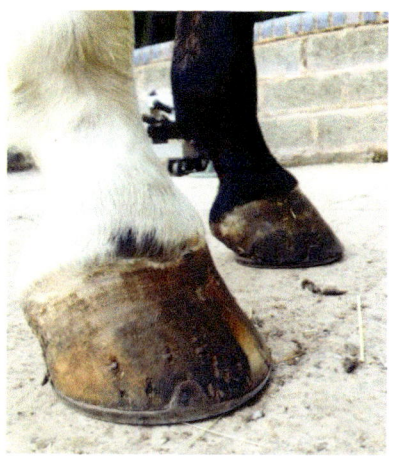

Grade 2 – The mismatch of the dorsal wall angle is 5-8° and diverging growth rings appear at the heel from the pull of the deep digital flexor tendon.

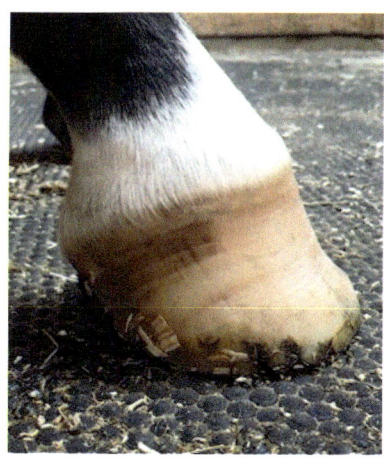

Grade 3 – The dorsal hoof wall has a dished appearance and bruising may appear on the sole from direct weight bearing.

Conditions involving hoof imbalance

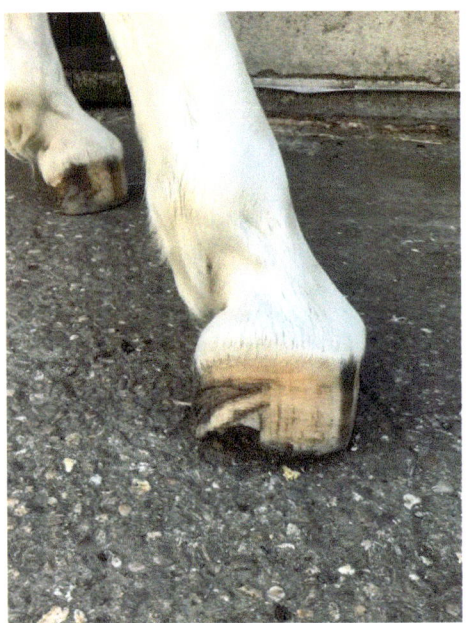

Grade 4 – The dorsal hoof wall angle is 80° or more with the sole supporting the weight of the bony column. The rear of the hoof has complete lack of function.

Treatment

Although much of the farriery treatment of club feet is preventing them from progressing into a higher grade, it is not possible to eradicate the condition in the adult horse and is more of a case of maintenance. Quite often there will be a medio-lateral imbalance due to the turned out appearance of the hoof with the upper limb opening out at the elbow. A lack of mass on the medial side of the solar surface of the hoof can be seen, so it is important to help establish a level footfall as possible. Heavily trimming down the heels is not advised as there is a high risk of creating a strain to the contracted deep digital flexor tendon and this can then result in lameness (O'Grady, 2012). However, by carefully lowering the heels during the trim so that there is some ground interaction for the frog will help to engage and utilise the deep digital flexor tendon (Fig. 6.14). Sometimes the use of a sole pack or graduated pad combined with shoes can be used to stimulate the rear third of the hoof, meaning that there will be less excessive heel growth at the next trim.

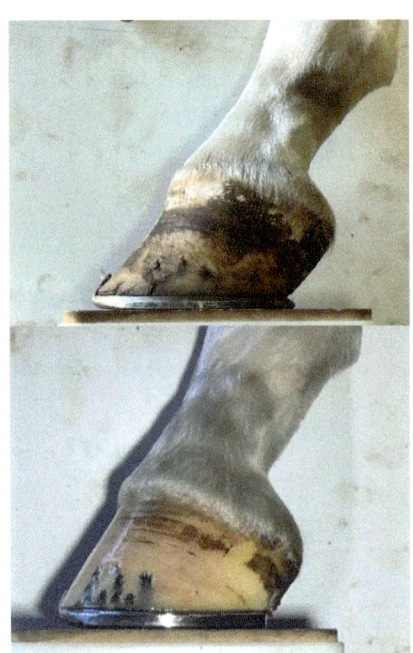

Fig. 6.14 Progress over time of a club foot that achieved a better hoof pastern alignment with careful trimming.

Hoof balance in relation to posture

The posture of the horse can play an important role in the balance of the feet (Fig. 6.15). There can be some discussion about what developed first in terms of poor hoof morphology and poor posture but often if one is corrected then the other follows suit (Sharp & Tabor, 2022).

Hoof balance affects the whole body with the protocols applied influencing the long term health of the horse. Assessing the horse on a flat, level concrete surface with all four feet stood square can give the best indication of any abnormalities (Kummer et al. 2006).

The range of conformational defects is described earlier in this book so this section will focus on the likely pathologies that can develop from acquired poor posture. A camped under posture behind can lead to collapsed heels, strain on the suspensory ligament, gluteal pain, inflammation to the sacroiliac (pelvis) joint and a negative plantar angle of the pedal bone (Fig. 6.16).

Some of this adapted posture can result in deviations of hoof flight where the landing phase of the stride being influenced by pain higher up (Fig. 6.17).

This acquired posture is likely to be corrected with hoof trimming and/or shoeing to achieve a normal hoof pastern axis. They may require the involvement of frog support as well as shoes fitted with sufficient length to overcome and adjust poor posture. The correction that takes place in the hoof should be combined with physiotherapist treatment due to the change in tension of the ascending limb and the muscles and fascia associated with it.

Repeat assessment of the horse's hoof balance and dynamic flight should be performed before trimming to ensure any minor defects can be addressed early.

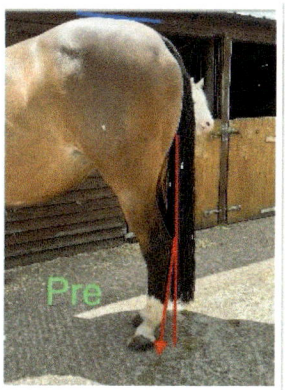
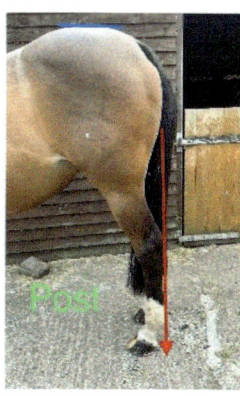

Fig. 6.15 Change in position of the cannon bone of the hind limb following a hoof trim combined with shoes fitted with plantar support.

Conditions involving hoof imbalance

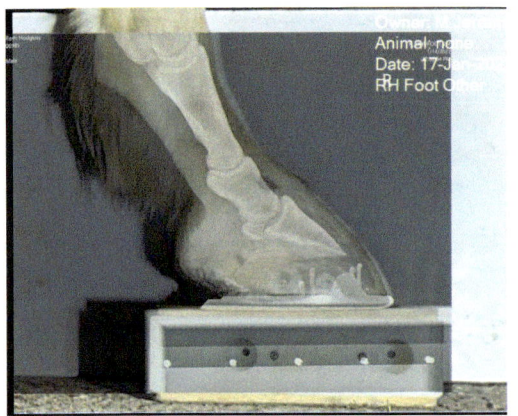

Fig. 6.16 A hoof with a negative plantar angle of the coffin bone as a result of compensating for sacro-iliac pain.

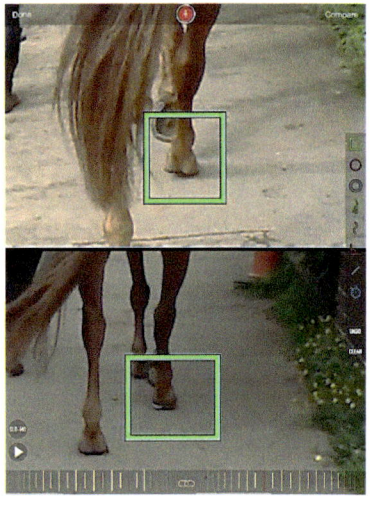

Fig. 6.17 Pain at the stifle area resulted in abnormal lateral first and secondary medial loading of the hind hoof. Post shoeing with a heart bar resulted in a much more even contact with the ground.

References

Caldwell, F. J. (2017) 'Flexural deformity of the distal interphalangeal joint' *Veterinary Clinics: Equine Practice*, Vol.33, No.2, pp 315-330.

Floyd, A. E. (2010) 'Use of a grading system to facilitate treatment and prognosis in horses with negative palmar angle syndrome (heel collapse): 107 cases' *Journal of Equine Veterinary Science*, Vol. 30, No,11, pp 666-675.

Hunt, R. J. (2012) 'Farriery for the hoof with low or underrun heels' *Veterinary Clinics of North America: Equine Practice*, Vol. 28, No.2, pp 351-364.

Kummer, M., Geyer, H., Imboden, I., Auer, J., & Lischer, C. (2006) 'The effect of hoof trimming on radiographic measurements of the front feet of normal Warmblood horses' *The Veterinary Journal*, Vol. 172, No.1, pp 58-66.

O'Grady, S. E., & Dryden, V. C. (2012) 'Farriery for the hoof with a high heel or club foot' *Veterinary Clinics: Equine Practice*, Vol. 28 No.2, pp 365-379.

Oosterlinck, M., Hardeman, L. C., Van Der Meij, B. R., Veraa, S., Van Der Kolk, J. H., Wijnberg, I. D., & Back, W. (2013) 'Pressure plate analysis of toe-heel and medio-lateral hoof balance at the walk and trot in sound sport horses' *The Veterinary Journal*, Vol. 198, pp e9-e13.

Sharp, Y., & Tabor, G. (2022) 'An Investigation into the Effects of Changing Dorso-Plantar Hoof Balance on Equine Hind Limb Posture' *Animals*, Vol. 12, No.23, pp 3275-3281.

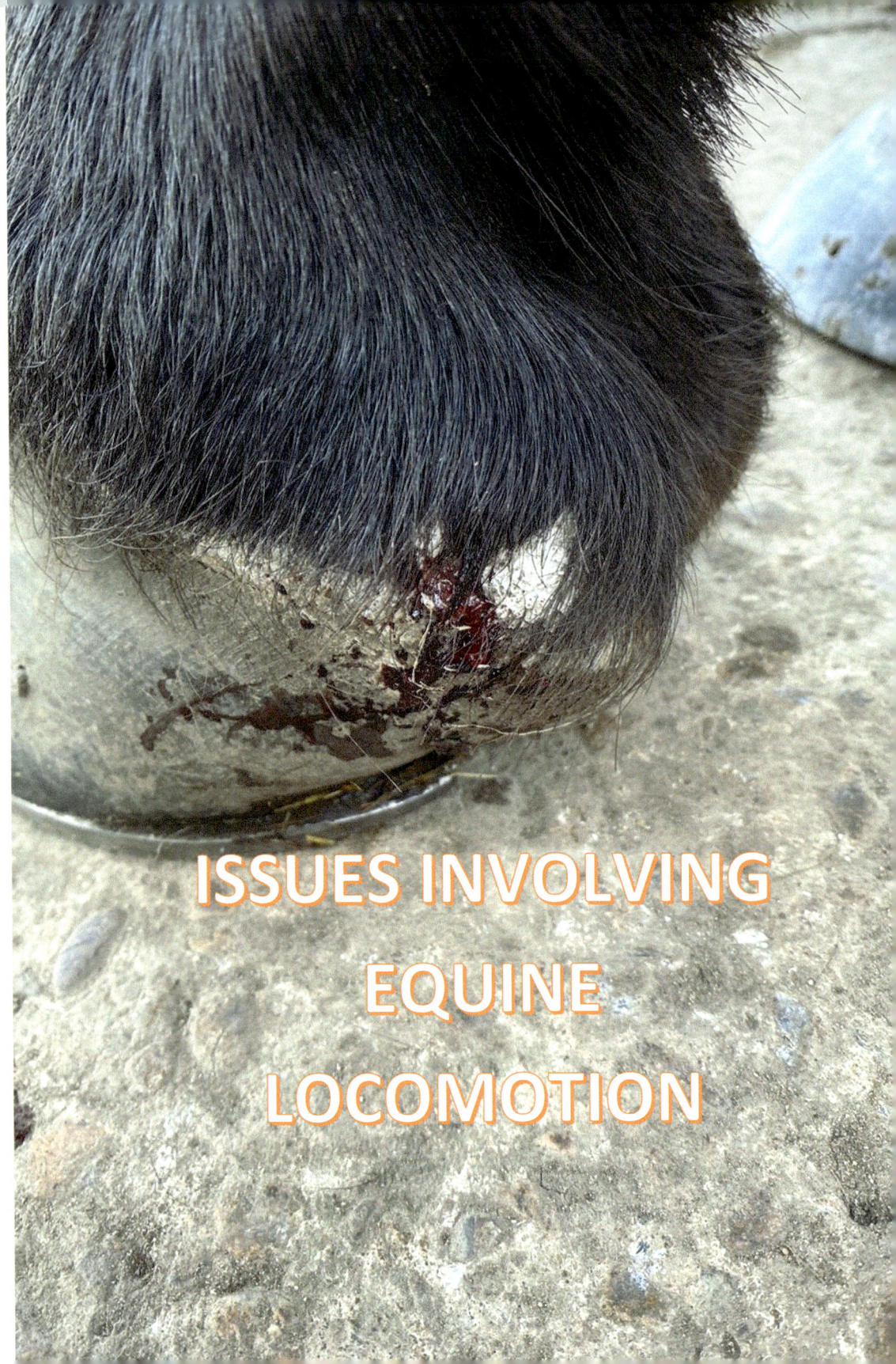

ISSUES INVOLVING EQUINE LOCOMOTION

Chapter 7 - Issues involving Equine Locomotion

Introduction

When the horse is moving either at any gait or speed, there is always a likelihood of collision with another limb or a change to the fluid motion of the swing phase of the stride. This can result in an abnormal injury occurring especially if the horse is starting to feel the effects of fatigue (Fig. 7.1).

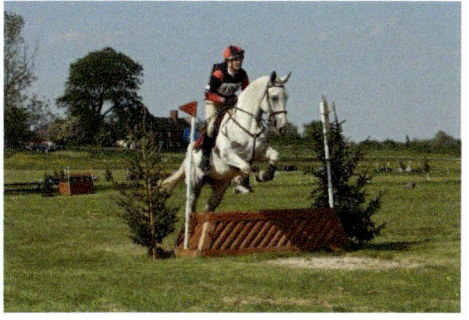

Fig 7.1 Fatigue can occur during the latter stages of a competition.

It is best practice to ensure the horse is fully warmed up before commencing faster work and that all tack and equipment is well fitted and in good working order. There also must be the consideration that the weight of the rider should be compared to the size of the horse and that it is humane to ride the horse even for light work.

Tripping/stumbling

Tripping occurs when the toe of the hoof stabs the ground causing the horse to propel forwards and, in some cases, bring the horse down completely. Quite often, fatigue plays a big part in tripping but can also be the result of a horse overdue for trimming and shoeing. A trim with a rounded toe edge can help to reduce the leverage upon the toe as forward propulsion and breakover takes place or a shoe can be applied with this mimicked in the toe profile (Fig. 7.2).

Ensure the horse is up to date with physiotherapy in case there is a pain compensation taking place elsewhere in the body leading to a lack of coordination between the limbs (Orlande et al. 2012). In extreme cases, knee boots may be required to prevent injury but that must only be a last option once other aspects have been evaluated by professionals.

Issues involving Equine Locomotion

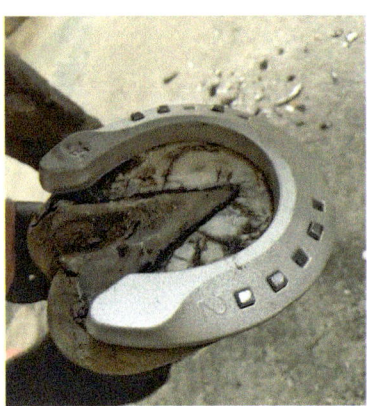

Fig. 7.2 A lightweight aluminium shoe that is heavy bevelled to help prevent tripping by ensuring a smooth and easy breakover of the hoof.

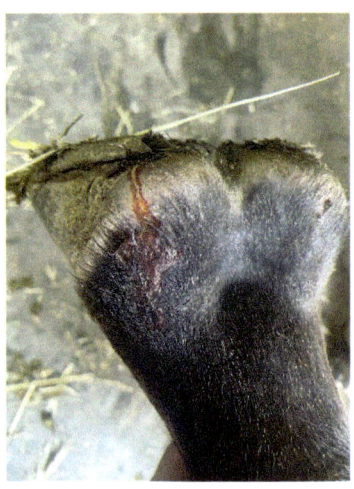

Fig. 7.3 Wound to the lateral heel bulb as a result of an overreach.

Overreach

An overreach occurs when a hind hoof collides with the heel bulbs or higher of a front hoof (Fig. 7.3). This can happen in both shod and unshod horses with the damage ranging from a minor blemish to an invasive avulsion. There are a few contributing factors to this occurring such as a poorly conformed horse (horses with a short coupled back), fatigue from prolonged periods of exercise, a failure to warm up correctly and long overgrown feet often resulting in a disoriented stride pattern.

Prevention of overreach injuries involves proper training and conditioning of the horse along with regular physiotherapist sessions to maintain strength and suppleness in the horse.

It is important to evaluate the likely cause before considering a treatment plan. The wound itself will need to be kept clean and dry with solutions such as diluted iodine being applied to eliminate bacteria and reduce the chances of infection developing. The use of overreach boots can help prevent future damage, but they must be fitted correctly to cover the heel bulbs in their entirety as the boots are likely to ride up the pastern during faster gaits (Fig. 7.4).

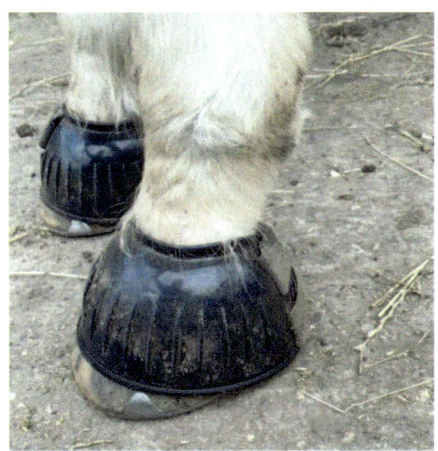

Fig. 7.4 A pair of well fitted overreach boots that protect the heels of the shoe and the rear of the hoof in its entirety.

hind hoof meaning there is less chance of collision (Fig. 7.5).

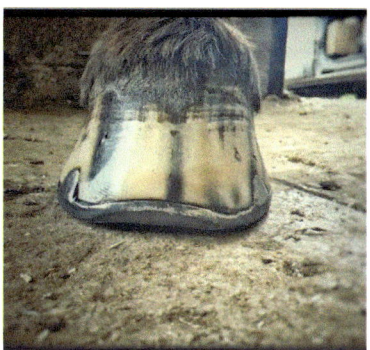

Fig. 7.5 A set toe fitted to a hind hoof. Note the folded up toe of the shoe to reduce the energy required for the hind foot to breakover. This also helps to alter the arc of flight so there is less chance of a collision with a front hoof.

Forging

Forging is when the toe of the hind hoof collides with the sole surface of the front foot most often at the toe or quarter. This can create a loud noise and is often associated with a fatigued horse or those that are overdue for a trim or shoes. This undesirable trait can also bring the horse down in extreme cases or lead to shoe loss.

Ensuring the horse is correctly warmed up before exercise can reduce the effects of this along with regular physiotherapy (Wang et al. 2021). Hind shoes can be fitted with a set toe or with extended heels to help alter the arc of flight of the

Brushing

Brushing is the act of a fore or hind limb colliding with the opposite limb. This happens more in the hind limb due to how close they are together and is exaggerated further if there is any pain in the hock or pelvis (Fig. 7.6).

Brushing tends to occur more in horses that are tired or have been worked for an extensive period (Horan at al. 2021). A lack of fitness and poor conformation such as base narrow or medial angular deviations of the lower limb are associated with excessive brushing. Quite

Issues involving Equine Locomotion

often the result is a scuffing of the hoof wall at the medial heel and in extreme cases can result in a wound or bleeding.

The use of sausage boots can help protect against coronary band brushing or if the interference is occurring above the fetlock, then well fitting brushing boots are recommended.

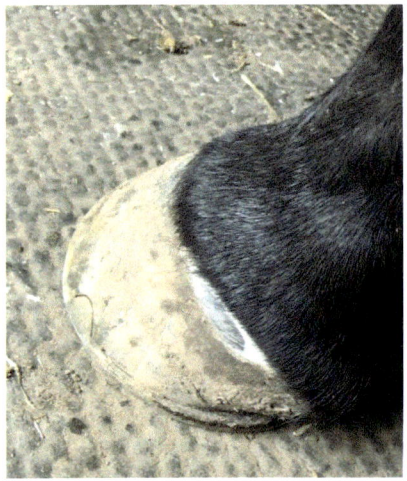

Fig. 7.6 A hoof showing scuff marks at the coronary band as a result of interference from the opposite limb.

Toe drag

A toe drag is when the hind feet square off and wear away at the toe due to lack of engagement of the hind end during riding (Fig. 7.7). This tends to happen in horses that are gaining their fitness and novice riders from not engaging the horses correctly. Toe drag can also be the result of pain in the proximal aspect of the suspensory ligament so it is important to establish the root cause before commencing any changes to trimming or shoeing as veterinary treatment may be required.

As a consequence of the shoe becoming thinner and weaker at the toe, the shoe can become "spread" by winging out past the perimeter of the hoof shape. This will result in the horse needed to be reshod and if there is excessive wear to the dorsal wall then a set toe shoe can be applied which was described in the forging section of this chapter.

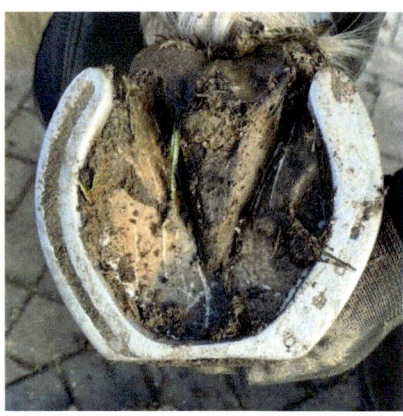

Fig. 7.7 A shoe that has excessively worn in the toe from dragging and has led to the shoe becoming spread.

Crossfire

Cross firing tends to occur mostly in harness racing horses when the hind foot collides with the diagonally opposite front limb and/or hoof (Moore, 2017). This is considered to be a very undesirable trait in standardbreds as it can slow down their pace or even bring the horse down. The hoof should be trimmed to establish a level footfall as possible in the hind feet with a trailer shoe applied to help orientate the hind hoof away from the midline as much as possible. Careful rounding of the medial aspect of the shoe can also enhance protection if collision were to occur (Fig. 7.8). The use of overreach boots can also be helpful during periods of exercise on the track at home.

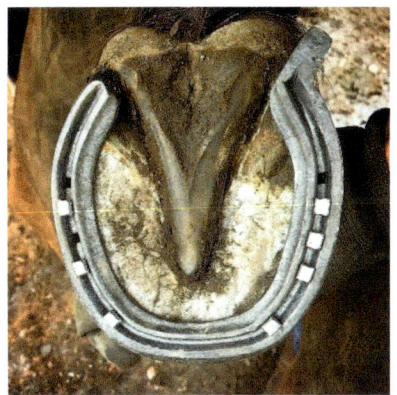

Fig. 7.8 A lightweight steel shoe with lateral trailer applied to a standardbred to help prevent crossfiring.

Slipping

Horses that work extensively on the road can be prone to slipping, particularly if the roads are overdue for resurfacing. This is predominantly an issue with shoes as barefoot hooves tend not to slip as much on the road. However, if the horse requires to wear shoes from excessive hoof wear or adjustment of conformational posture, it is possible to apply tungsten pins or road nails to provide sufficient grip (Fig. 7.9).

These protrude around a millimetre above the ground surface of the shoe to provide grip with the tungsten steel having strong grip properties and ideally fitted with one on each heel to prevent rocking of the hoof during the stance phase (Day et al. 2020).

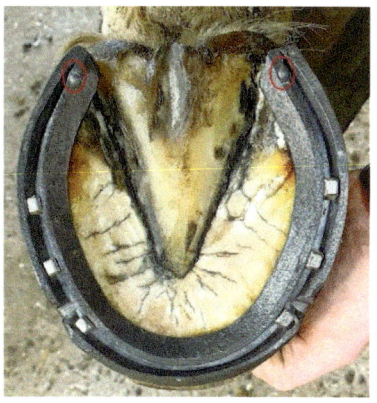

Fig. 7.9 A pair of tungsten pins (circled) driven in the shoe towards the heel following drilling of a pilot hole post fitting.

Additional grip can take place with drive in plug studs or calkins but these should be fitted with caution as they can have a detrimental effect to the structures at the rear third of the hoof due to the increased elevation off the ground.

A traditional roadster shoe with the height of the toe matching the heights of the heels provide less damage but still lead to a lack of ground interaction with the hoof (Fig. 7.10)

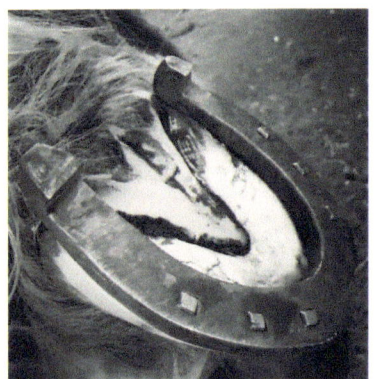

Fig. 7.10 A plain stamped calkin and wedge shoe for a carriage horse that worked on cobbled roads.

If a horse is to compete on grass, then the application of screw in studs can be beneficial to increase grip on uneven and varying ground. These can be screwed before the competitive round and removed as soon as the class has finished. Most studs used now are 10mm diameter with 8mm studs being phased out, so it is important to purchase the correct size stud relative to the holes punched in the shoes (Fig. 7.11 and 7.12).

There is much debate about whether to apply one or two studs to a horse when competing (Lesniak & Gibson 2019). Whilst it is without question the horse will be more evenly balanced with bilateral studs, there is also the danger of a tread injury to the opposite limb with the medial stud especially with young horses who are still to establish their gait.

Each horse is unique so a judgement should take place on the horse's experience, type of going, quality of the course and the likelihood of fatigue. The smallest studs should be used as possible in relation to the cut in the ground in order to prevent "over braking" of the limb.

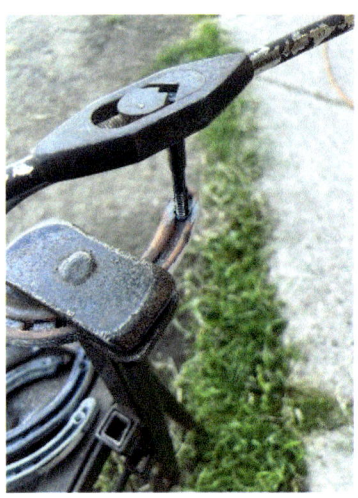

Fig. 7.11 Threading a stud hole using a 10mm tap following shoe fitting.

Issues involving Equine Locomotion

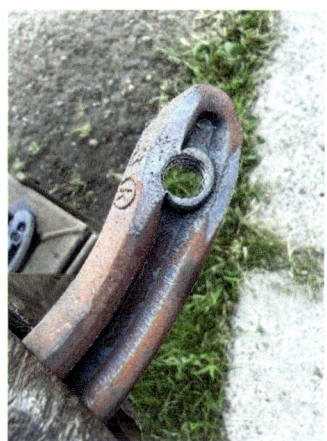

Fig. 7.12 Stud holes punched and threaded ready to complete the shoeing process.

The process of applying a stud for competition

Once the stud holes have been applied by the farrier and shoeing has completed, it is recommended that the holes are plugged with a suitable material that can be easily removed when arriving a competition. Below is a step by step guide on how to apply studs to shoes.

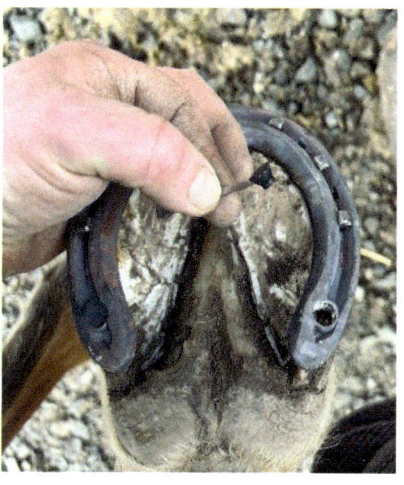

1. Remove the packing with a horseshoe nail.

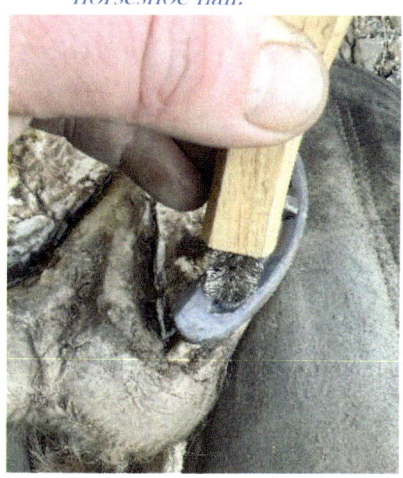

2. Clean out the hole using a small wire brush.

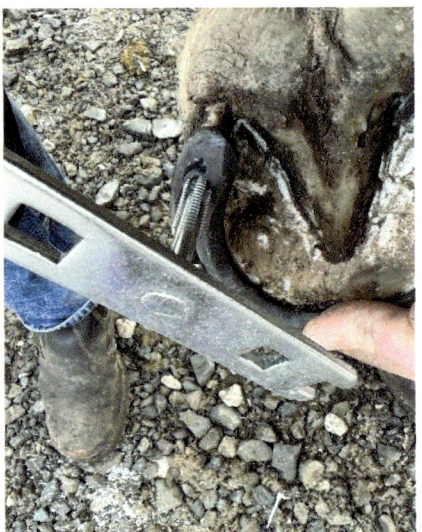

3. If required, rethread the hole using a 3/8" or 10mm threaded tap.

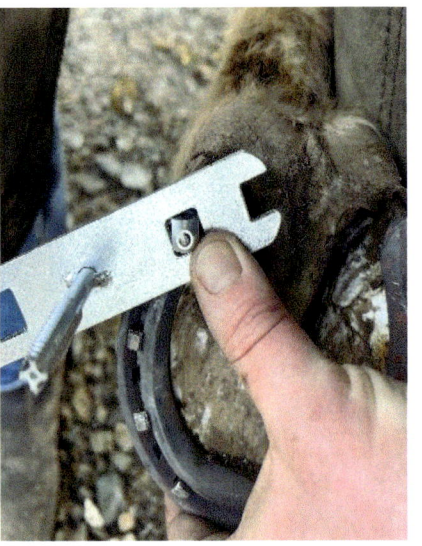

5. Using the spanner, tighten the stud so the shoulder is flush with the surface of the shoe.

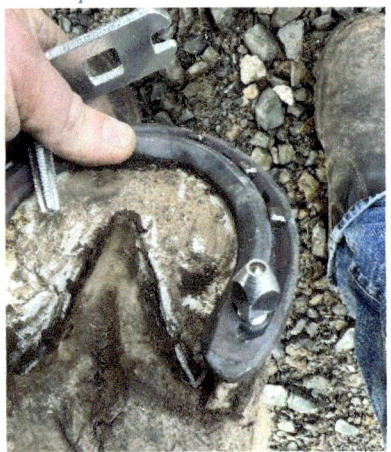

4. Hand tighten the stud in a clockwise direction.

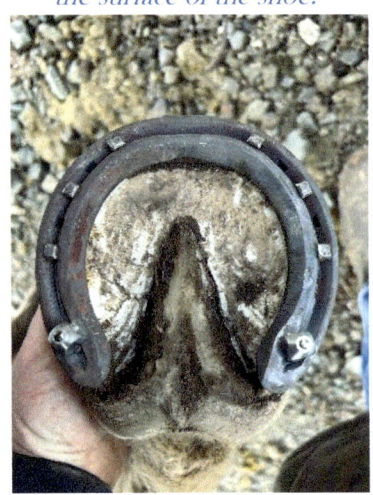

6. Repeat the process on the opposite side and the horse is ready for work.

References

Day, P., Collins, L., Horan, K., Weller, R., & Pfau, T. (2020) 'The Effect of Tungsten Road Nails on Upper Body Movement Asymmetry in Horses Trotting on Tarmac' *Journal of equine veterinary science*, Vol. 90, pp 103-110.

Horan, K., Kourdache, K., Coburn, J., Day, P., Brinkley, L., Carnall, H., & Pfau, T. (2021) 'Jockey perception of shoe and surface effects on hoof-ground interactions and implications for safety in the galloping thoroughbred racehorse' *Journal of Equine Veterinary Science*, Vo. 97, pp 103-127.

Lesniak, K., & Gibson, A. (2019). The Effect of Heel Studs on Retraction Kinematics of the Equine Hind-limb during Canter on Grass. In *9th Alltech-Hartpury Student Conference*.

Orlande, O., Hobbs, S. J., Martin, J. H., Owen, A. G., & Northrop, A. J. (2012) 'Measuring hoof slip of the leading limb on jump landing over two different equine arena surfaces' *Comparative exercise physiology*, Vol.8, No.1, pp 33-39.

Moore, W. J. (2017). *Balancing and Shoeing Trotting and Prancing Horses*. Read Books Ltd: Redditch

Wang, P., Takawira, C., Taguchi, T., Niu, X., Nazzal, M. D., & Lopez, M. J. (2021) 'Assessment of the effect of horseshoes with and without traction adaptations on the gait kinetics of nonlame horses during a trot on a concrete runway' *American Journal of Veterinary Research*, Vol.82, No.4, pp 292-301.

CONDITIONS OF THE SOFT TISSUES

Chapter 8 - Conditions of the soft tissues

Introduction

The soft tissues of the body make up the connections between the bones and provide the power to move the skeletal system. The soft tissues of the hoof involve the ligaments, tendons, bursae, cartilages, corium and other shock absorbing structures that cannot be evaluated by radiography. They assist in locomotion of the horse, prevent hyper extension or flexion of the limb and hoof to use energy in an efficient way.

A tendon is a fibrous cord by a way of muscle being attached to bone and are divided into flexor (back of the limb) or extensor (front of the limb) that either flex or extend the limb (Fig. 8.1). There are no muscles below the knee, the flexor and extensor tendons have muscular heads at the proximal aspect of the forelimb skeleton. Tendons have high tensile strength whilst being elastic and are capable of absorbing and storing energy.

A ligament is a band of fibrous tissue that connects bone or cartilage. Ligaments hold joints, bones and other structures together to provide stability to the limb. Ligaments tend to have less stretch and elasticity to the tendons as they are much shorter and stiffer than tendons. Ligaments also have greater resistance to forces of torque shearing and twisting than tendons.

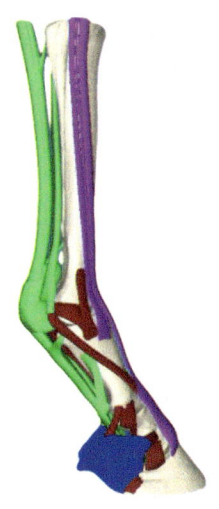

Fig. 8.1 The ligaments and tendons that flex (green) and extend (purple) the lower limb. The collateral ligaments (brown) provide stability to the joints whilst the collateral cartilages (blue) absorb concussion*.

Soft tissue injuries are a relatively common cause of lameness in the athletic horse. These injuries can be

Conditions of the soft tissues

difficult to diagnose, manage, and can take considerable time for complete healing to occur (Al-Agele et al. 2019). Injury to these soft tissues can occur as a result of trauma or mechanical overload as well as fatigue. Injury then occurs as a result of the fibre bundles becoming stretched beyond their capacity and rupture. These ruptured fibre bundles then fill with fluid and the inflammatory response begins.

Injury can occur from a singular catastrophic event or repeated low grade fibre ruptures that eventually become a large scale inflammatory response. The correct term for a tendon injury is a strain whilst a ligament injury is referred to as a sprain.

Due to the inability of radiography to diagnose soft tissue injury, it is usually advisable to investigate using **MRI**, ultrasound or CT scans in order to establish the damage sustained.

Collateral ligament injury

Collateral ligaments are found either side of a joint and there are many sets in the lower limb, but the most common injury occurs to the collateral ligament of the coffin joint. This usually happens on uneven ground causing one side of the joint to overextend and strain the ligament attached reducing its efficiency in stabilisation (Abu-Seida & Elmmawy, 2021).

This is also common in horses with lower limb deviations such as fetlock valgus and varus, this is due to the increased chance of unlevel footfall creating a repetitive strain on either side of a joint (Fig. 8.2). The injury is diagnosed using **MRI** with box rest advised for at least 3 months (Beasley et al. 2020).

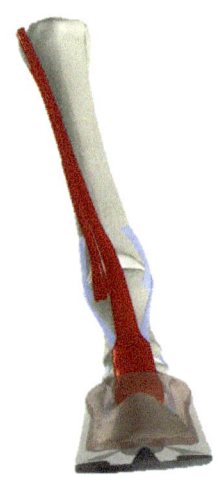

Fig. 8.2 Uneven loading of the hoof can result in straining the collateral ligament on the side of the joint experiencing the most torsion.

Treatment

Veterinary treatment involves the use of non-steroidal anti-inflammatory drugs for pain relief. Some cases may involve Interluekin Receptor Antagonist Protein (IRAP) treatment to reduce inflammation and encourage joint healing. There are some cases where shoes are removed, and the horse is kept barefoot during recovery. Wide branch shoes can be applied in some cases to help spread load of the effected side over a greater surface area (Fig. 8.3).

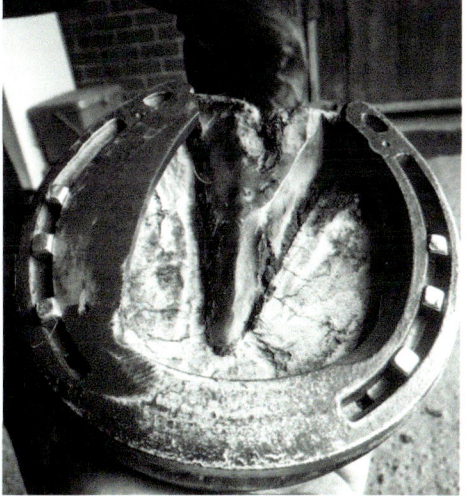

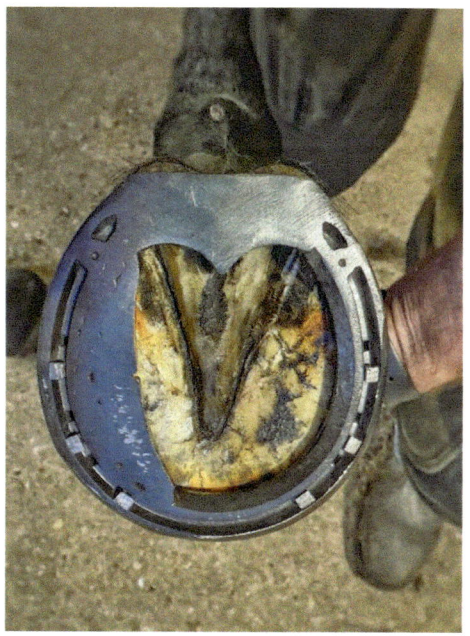

Fig. 8.4 A wide medial branch bar shoe applied for a horse with a medial collateral ligament sprain.

Fig. 8.3 A wide medial branch shoe, note the concavity of the lateral branch.

The author has found mild success with these shoes and has had better results using a wide webbed straight bar shoe, particularly for those with conformational faults and/or a poor medio-lateral balance (Fig. 8.4).

Deep digital flexor tendon injury

A deep digital flexor tendon injury tends to occur in horses with low heels and a broken back hoof pastern axis. This is due to the overload of the structures at the rear of the hoof during impact and mid stance especially if the horse starts to feel fatigued (Fig. 8.5).

Conditions of the soft tissues

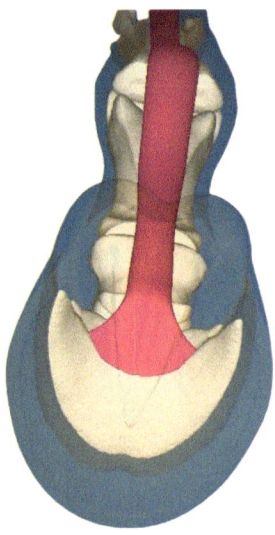

Fig. 8.5 The deep digital flexor tendon (pink) as it passes over the navicular bone before making a wide fanned out insertion onto the semi lunar crescent of the distal phalanx*.

There will be a large swelling in some cases where the strain has taken place higher up towards the fetlock but there can be minimal to no swelling if the injury has taken place in the hoof close to the insertion point (Cillán-García et al. 2013). For injuries within the hoof, an MRI will be required for an accurate diagnosis and to confirm the severity of the injury.

Treatment

The horse will require to be kept on box rest for a prolonged period whilst the damaged tendon recovers. Removing shoes and keeping barefoot is functional for many cases during the recovery period but there are also horses that would benefit from heel elevation to reduce tension in the damaged tendon (Hewitt-Dedman et al. 2022). This can take the form of a graduated bar shoe or pad, but it is advised to fit these with frog support to prevent descend of the frog and heel bulbs through the shoeing package (Fig. 8.6).

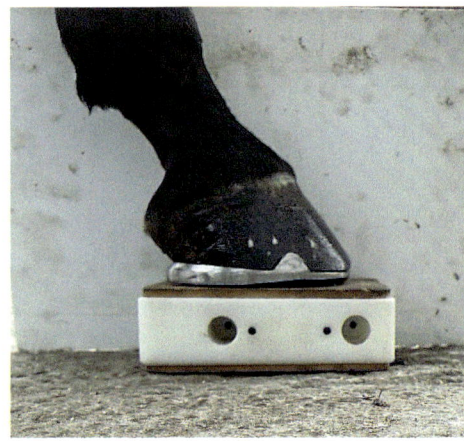

Fig. 8.6 A graduated bar shoe applied to a horse with a deep digital flexor tendon injury.

Prognosis is often guarded for a return to full pre injury performance but less severe cases have a better chance providing a careful recovery plan has been followed.

Conditions of the soft tissues

Soft tissue injury

Soft tissue injuries in the hoof can present as a mild to severe lameness depending on the location and the damage caused. Quite often there will be hardly any symptoms present such as swelling or increased pulse or heat. These injuries present worse when worked on a circle or on hard ground.

This can include sprain or rupture of the smaller ligaments found within the lower limb and hoof along with bone bruising which is sometimes referred to as a pedal bone oedema (Holroyd et al. 2013).

These cases benefit from a long period of rest to allow inflammation to subside and repair of the ligament. The use of frog support pads and shoes applied with leverage reduction can assist both those on rest and beginning light work (Fig. 8.7). This helps for two reasons – firstly to help realign the internal structures of the hoof to help prevent future recurrence and secondly to offer protection to the damaged area. This can also be achieved in the barefoot horse providing the original injury was from a single trauma incident rather than repetitive strain over a long period on a disfunctional hoof.

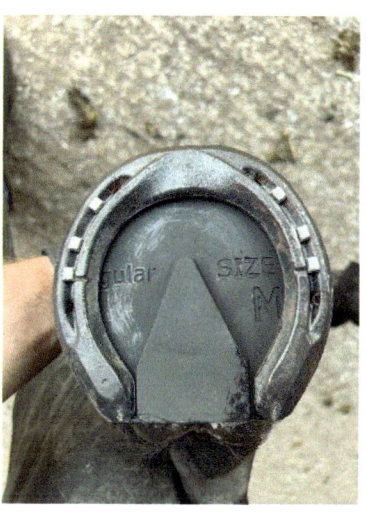

Fig. 8.7 A part leather, part synthetic frog support pad applied to a horse with a pedal bone oedema.

Once recovery has been achieved, care and consideration for the horse's working surface must be considered (Ross & Dyson, 2010). Horses will perform better on some surfaces more than others and that is down to the individual horse's way of going. Filming your horses working on a particular surface will help to identify their comfort levels and how willing they are to work. When it comes to competing on a grass surface, ensure the arena is well prepared and is flat and level. Do not risk a repeat injury if the ground is excessively hard or soft, it is much preferable to wait or compete at another venue.

References

Abu-Seida, A. M., & Elemmawy, Y. M. (2021) 'Chronic Collateral Sesamoidean Desmopathy in Draft Horses: Magnetic Resonance Imaging and Histopathological Findings' *Journal of Equine Veterinary Science*, Vol. 98, pp 103-122.

Al-Agele, R., Paul, E., Dvojmoc, V. K., Sturrock, C. J., Rauch, C., & Rutland, C. S. (2019) 'The anatomy, histology and physiology of the healthy and lame equine hoof' *Veterinary Anatomy and Physiology*, Vol. 13.

Beasley, B., Selberg, K., Giguère, S., & Allen, K. (2020) 'Magnetic resonance imaging characterisation of lesions within the collateral ligaments of the distal interphalangeal joint – 28 cases' *Equine Veterinary Education*, Vol. 32, pp 11-17.

Cillán-García, E., Milner, P. I., Talbot, A., Tucker, R., Hendey, F., Boswell, J., & Taylor, S. E. (2013) 'Deep digital flexor tendon injury within the hoof capsule; does lesion type or location predict prognosis?' *Veterinary Record*, Vol. 173, No.3, pp 70-80.

Gray, P. (1994) '*Lameness*' London: JA Allen.

Hewitt-Dedman, C. L., Biggi, M., Van Zadelhoff, C., Schwarz, T., Reardon, R. J. M., & Taylor, S. E. (2022) 'Imaging findings and clinical outcome of foot pain attributable to insertional deep digital flexor tendon injury and/or fluid signal within the flexor surface of the distal phalanx' *Equine Veterinary Education*, Vol. 34, No.10, e422-e430.

Holroyd, K., Dixon, J. J., Mair, T., Bolas, N., Bolt, D. M., David, F., & Weller, R. (2013) 'Variation in foot conformation in lame horses with different foot lesions' *The Veterinary Journal*, Vol. 195, No.3, pp 361-365.

Ross, M. W., & Dyson, S. J. (2010) '*Diagnosis and Management of Lameness in the Horse*' Elsevier Health Sciences: London.

* Images adapted with kind permission from Effigos AG. Hoof Explorer

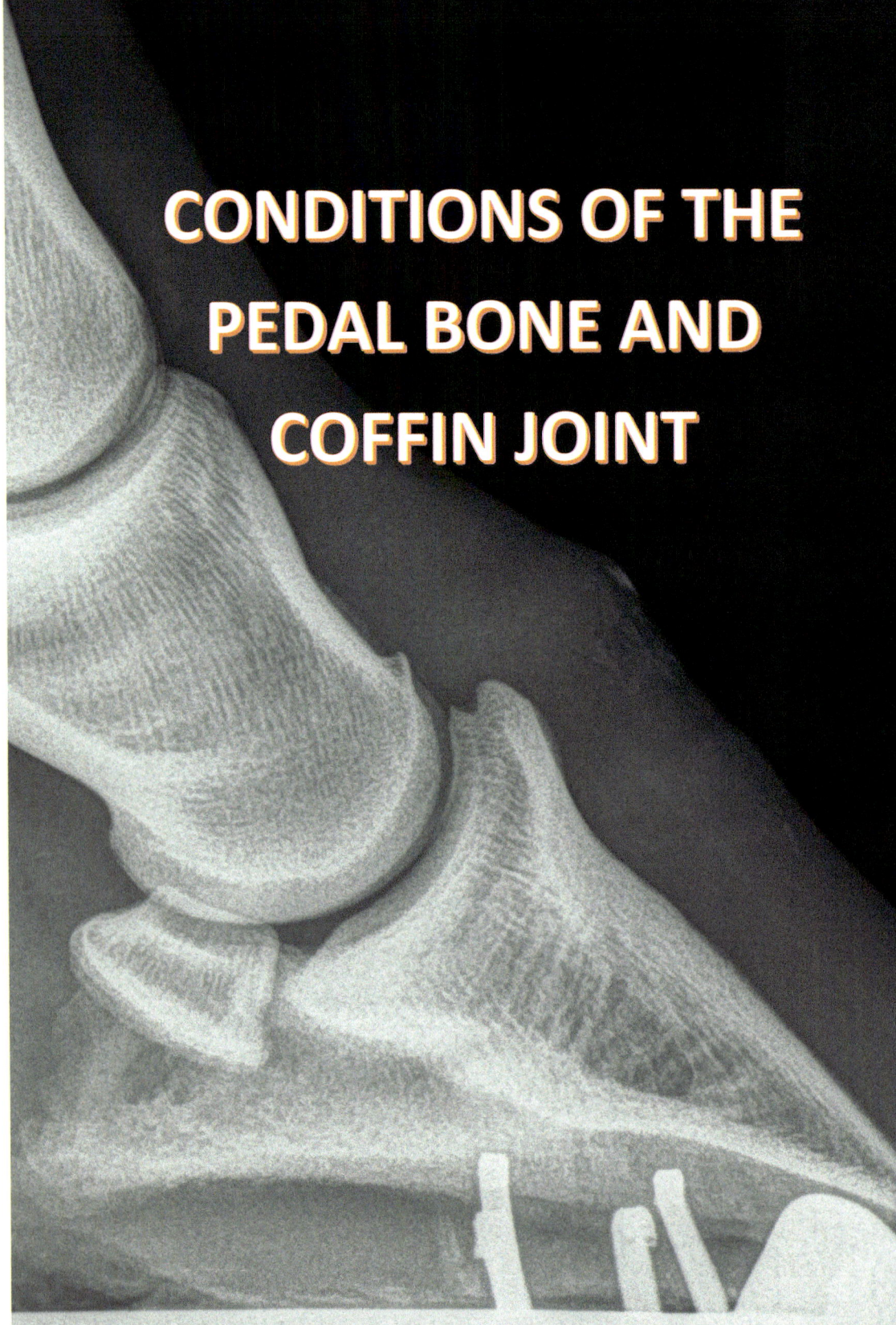

CONDITIONS OF THE PEDAL BONE AND COFFIN JOINT

Conditions of the Pedal Bone and Coffin Joint

Chapter 9 - Conditions of the pedal bone and coffin joint

Introduction

The coffin joint is made up of the distal extremity of the middle phalanx (short pastern) bone, the proximal extremity of the distal phalanx (coffin or pedal bone) and the dorsal surface of the distal sesamoid (navicular bone). The coffin joint is found within the hoof and is a composite synovial joint which means it is made up of more than 2 bones (Fig. 9.1). The coffin bone resembles the shape of the hoof by which it is enclosed.

The structural design is composed of dense cortical bone with a small cavity known as the semi lunar sinus which is where digital arteries converge. The coffin bone is covered by vascular tissue and blood vessels which is known as the sensitive foot. The shape of the coffin bone differs in front and hind feet due to the primary function of weight bearing on fore limbs with a more vaulted and pointed shape in hind feet for the purpose of propulsion.

The distal sesamoid (navicular bone) is covered with a small plate of complimentary fibro-cartilage which provides a gliding surface for the deep digital flexor tendon to pass over. There is a bursa located between the navicular bone and deep digital flexor tendon known as the navicular bursa which releases synovial fluid to help keep the joint lubricated.

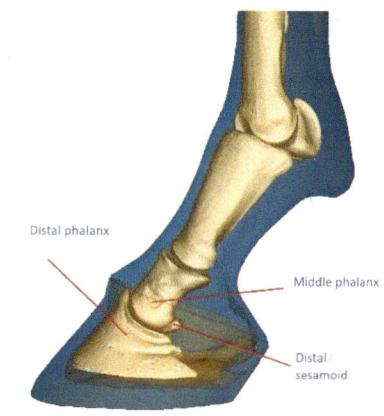

Fig. 9.1 The composition of the coffin joint. *

Laminitis

Laminitis is described as an inflammation of the dermal laminae of the hoof. As the laminae suspend the horse's bodyweight within the hoof, when it begins to fail and separate, the pedal bone can rotate in response to pain

141

with contraction of the deep digital flexor tendon. In some cases, the bony column can sink in the hoof with a chance the pedal bone can then penetrate through the protective sole underneath (Pollitt, 2004). There will be considerable lameness present with an increased digital pulse found at the fetlock along with heat present on the hoof wall (Fig. 9.2).

A strong response is noted when hoof testers are pressed on the sole as well as a reluctance to bear weight on the opposite limb whilst holding a hoof in the air for investigation (Fig 9.3). A reluctance to turn or move backwards can be present as well as deep stressed breathing.

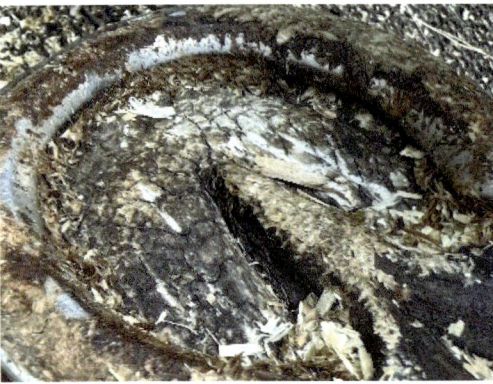

Fig. 9.2 A thin tender sole that can flex to thumb pressure is often evident.

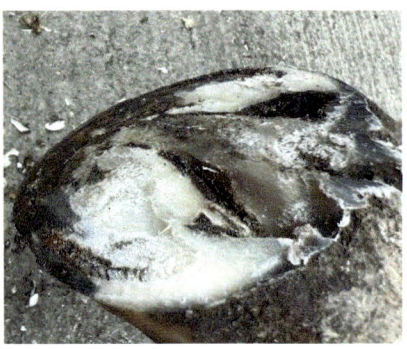

Fig. 9.3 Dropped soles are common with horses that have suffered a laminitic episode.

It goes without saying that Laminitis is one of the most common killers of horses and should be treated as urgently as colic.

Emergency first aid when a case of Laminitis is suspected.

1. Bring the horse in on box rest with a deep shavings or sand bed that covers the entirety of the stable.
2. Contact the veterinarian immediately and they will come out to examine the horse's heart rate, provide pain relief by intravenous and/or oral administration and condition score the horse.
3. It is advised not to remove shoes or trim horses at the early stages due to the instability of the laminae, this could make the condition far worse. This also counts for horses that are overdue a farriery visit.

4. The farrier or vet can apply a frog support to the hoof, this can be as simple as an offcut of EVA rubber, frog support pad or impression material. Do not load the front half of the hoof due to the danger of creating a pressure point with the tip of the pedal bone (Fig. 9.4).
5. Access to hay should be provided and the horse should not be starved. (hay feeding techniques described below).
6. Maintain a calm environment for the horse that is on box rest by leaving another horse in view and by creating minimal disruption around the yard.

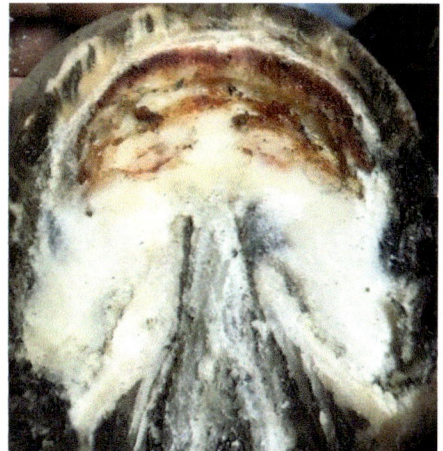

Fig. 9.4 Damage to the sole as a result of the pedal rotating.

Feeding hay for laminitics

Hay should be fed as a maximum of 1.5% of the horse's bodyweight per day when measured as dry matter. This should be split between morning and night. For horses that eat their hay at a fast rate then the use of double netting can slow down the consumption rate.

It is recommended that the hay is analysed using a laboratory equine forage analysis to determine the Non Structural Carbohydrate (NSC) level by adding together the Water Soluble Carbohydrate (WSC) and starch percentiles.

NSC refers to sugar, starch and fructan levels which create an insulin spike in the horse's body. These should be under 10% for laminitic horses, a mixed meadow hay is preferred due to the lower NSC level. Hay should be soaked for an hour with hot water followed by an hour with cold water, this will help to bring the NSC level down to around 5% in most types of hay.

Hay that is soaked longer than this period will become less palatable along with vital nutrients leached during the soaking process. This can result in horses requiring a balancer in order to meet the daily foundational nutritional requirements of the horse.

A deep stable bed made up of shavings or sand is advised to help stabilise the arch of sole, this can also be further enhanced with a frog support pad and/or packing applied to the sole in the rear half of the hoof only. Laminitis cases are broken down into categories dependant on the cause and the treatment response required.

Endocrinopathic laminitis

This refers to a hormone response in the body and the subsequent reaction in the hooves. The two most common types are Equine Metabolic Syndrome (EMS) and Pituitary Pars Intermedia Dysfunction (PPID) also referred to as Cushing's disease.

Equine Metabolic Syndrome

EMS is the result of insulin disregulation in the horse often characterised with a thick cresty neck and an overweight appearance. Insulin is a hormone produced by the pancreas which found in the abdomen around 2 feet behind the girth area on the off side of the horse. About 98% of the pancreas produces enzymes that break down food and the remaining 2% produces hormones such as insulin that help carbohydrate, protein and fat to breakdown products that enter the cells.

Insulin levels peak in the morning and gradually lower throughout the day. EMS is the inability to respond to and use the insulin produced by the body because the insulin is not functioning properly, and as a result the blood glucose is not moving into the cells as it usually does.

The pancreas then senses that the original increased output is not working so therefore increases the amount of insulin. Typically, the main characteristic of insulin resistance is high insulin and normal glucose.

In early insulin resistance you may see four or five times the amount of insulin being developed to allow for glucose to be controlled (Johnson et al. 2010). Blood tests are performed to monitor the insulin level with a medication such as Levothyroxine a possibility should the horse not respond enough to dietary changes (Fig. 9.5).

Horses that have insulin resistance can often develop Equine Metabolic Syndrome (EMS) and consequently laminitis. These horses often have an obese appearance, flat soles, stretched white lines with bruising present on the sole (Fig. 9.6). Significant changes to the diet and management will be required to lower insulin levels, sugar intake and eventually substantial weight loss.

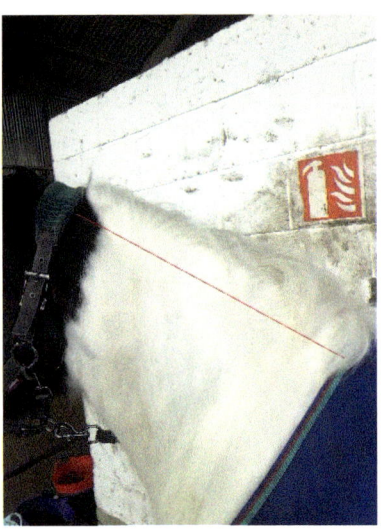

Fig. 9.5 A recovering laminitic horse with a cresty neck. The excess above the red line indicates a disregulation of insulin. If the crest is stiff and immobile, then the condition is at an advanced stage.

Conditions of the Pedal Bone and Coffin Joint

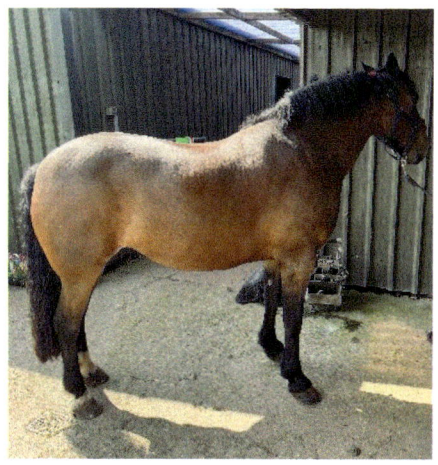

Fig. 9.6 Other clinical signs of insulin resistance include fat deposits at the shoulders and croup along with a flat surface area on the top of the back.

Pituitary Pars Intermedia Disfunction

Pituitary Pars Intermedia Disfunction (PPID) or Cushing's disease is a hormonal condition arising from the pituitary gland and creating changes throughout the whole body. In PPID, the normal mechanisms which control hormone production by the pituitary gland are damaged and the inhibitory part becomes lost. Thus, there is excessive production of the normal hormones from the pituitary gland. These hormones then enter the circulation and affect the whole body.

A well-recognised symptom of PPID is the appearance of a thick curly coat, however this occurs in much more advanced cases and there are many other subtle symptoms that can be picked up on earlier (Fig. 9.7). Most obvious signs are a change in coat condition, filling around the eyes, excessive drinking and urination along with a reduction in the body's defence system resulting in infections or abscesses. There will also be abnormal deposits of fat above the eyes, withers, sheath and croup.

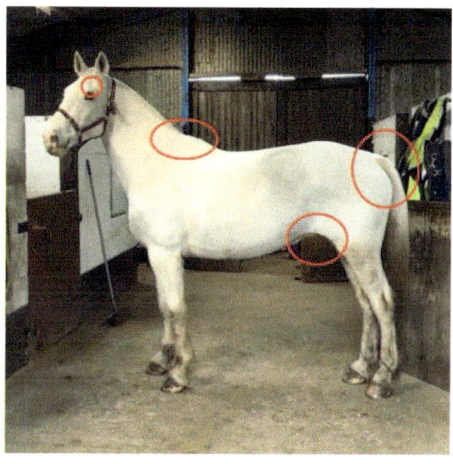

Fig. 9.7 The red circled areas highlight where fatty deposits develop with PPID.

PPID will require blood test diagnostics to monitor the Adreno corticotropic hormone (ACTH) level with treatment as necessary with pergolide medication, in most circumstances a reading of 40 pg/ml (picograms per millilitre) or below is considered to be negative for PPID. However, this level can vary depending on the type of test used and time of year, so it is best to consult with a veterinarian when assessing the findings. For some horses that have the symptoms of PPID but test negative to blood testing then the use of a Thyrotropin Releasing Hormone (TRH) stimulation test can help to detect horses that may require medication.

However, there are some horses that do not respond well to the medication with a loss of condition, depression and discomfort. If this is the case, consider using herbal remedies such as agnus castus to help control the condition.

Trauma induced Laminitis

Laminitis can be brought on by repetitive and excessive concussion to the hooves (also known as road founder) as well as response to a traumatic incident (such as being stuck in a gate). There may some argument that the horse already some clinical symptoms prior to the trauma incident that may have tipped the horse into full blown laminitis. It is imperative with these cases that the horse is kept settled during the recovery phase, this can be helped by bringing in a horse to keep them company and creating minimal disruption on the yard.

Supporting limb laminitis

Supporting limb laminitis refers to an overload of a single limb as a result of attempting to take weight off an opposite limb. This can happen when horses suffer a significant tendon injury or bone fracture and consequently, bear the weight of both limbs on a single limb (Fig. 9.8).

Due to this overload, the blood supply to the laminae becomes compromised and the ability to suspend the horse's bodyweight becomes inhibited (Van Eps et al. 2010).

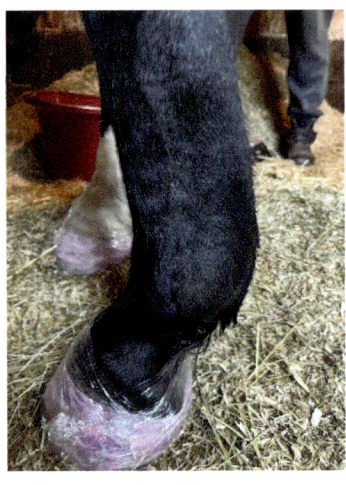

Fig. 9.8 A suspensory ligament injury to the left forelimb of this horse caused an overload on the opposite limb resulting in supporting limb laminitis.

Toxaemia

This refers to a toxic reaction in the body to a foreign mass in the blood and lymphatic system. This includes brood mares that have retained the afterbirth post foaling or horses that have eaten poisonous feed such as chicken feed. There are limited studies that suggest that steroids can induce laminitis, but it is more likely to be a cortisol reaction and many of these horses have undiagnosed EMS or PPID present.

In these cases, toxins are produced by bacteria that have entered the bloodstream through the hindgut, wound or other infection site. The reaction in the hindgut leads to acidosis and subsequently the horse develops laminitis.

Hoof sloughing

This refers to when a poor response to the original laminitic incident has resulted in a separation at the coronary band with the likelihood the hoof will come off (Fig. 9.9). There are cases where this can be resolved by keeping horses upright in a harness until a new hoof has grown but in the author's opinion, this is not humane, and the kindest thing is euthanasia with these cases.

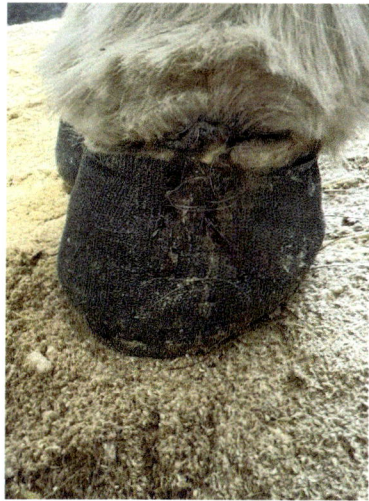

Fig. 9.9 An example of a hoof about to slough. The coronary band is bleeding and separating from the skin above.

Radiography for laminitis

A well taken set of radiographs are vital for accurate and successful treatment of laminitis. The two most critical views are the latero-medial (LM) projection and the dorso-palmar (DP) projection for determining the position of the pedal bone and the bony column along with the degree of rotation of the pedal bone and if any medial sinkage has taken place.

A steel marker should be applied to the top of the hoof in line with the coronary band for the LM projection to help assess the amount of sinkage of the pedal bone, this is also known as the founder distance (Fig. 9.10). It should be noted that very horses have a zero founder distance even when healthy, therefore a distance of 0.9cm or more is considered significant with the chances of a successful outcome becoming reduced as the distance increases.

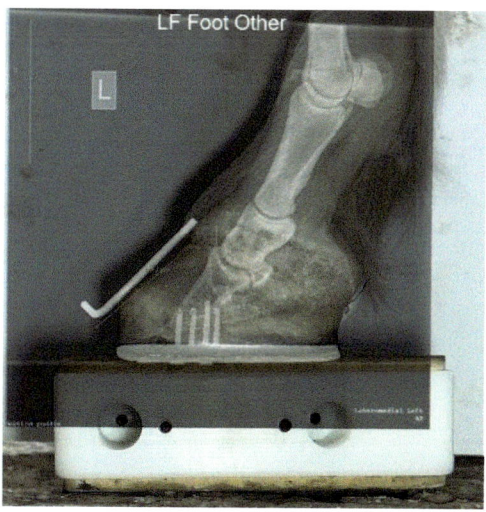

Fig. 9.10 A LM radiograph superimposed on a lateral photograph. Note the steel marker on the hoof wall.

Types of Founder

Type 1 founder

A type 1 founder hoof has low weak heels, a flat soles and an overexpansion of the hoof wall and white line (Fig. 9.11). In some of these cases there is minimal rotation of the coffin bone but a marked descent of the bony column within the hoof.

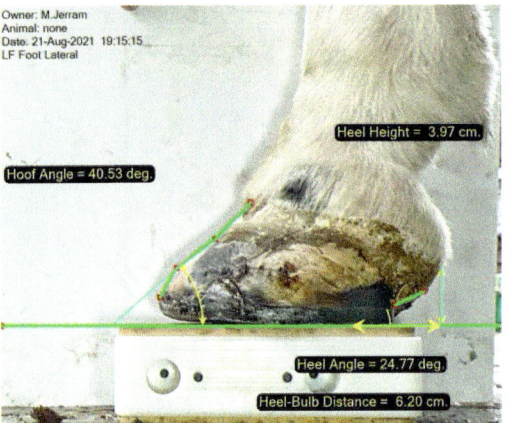

Fig. 9.11 A type 1 founder with a distorted coronary band.

Type 2 founder

A type 2 founder has a considerable amount of heel growth, diverging growth rings and a long distorted toe (Fig. 9.12). This is often associated with rotation of the coffin bone and in some cases, there is also sinkage of the bony column.

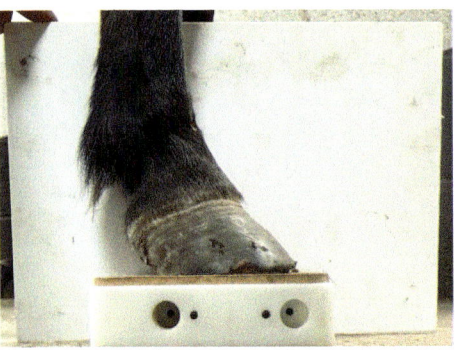

Fig. 9.12 An example of a type 2 foundered hoof with excessive heel and distorted toe.

Treatment

Veterinary treatment of laminitis will involve the use of non-steroidal anti-inflammatory drugs to provide pain relief during the early stages. In some cases, the use of paracetamol or Acepromazine (ACP) can also be administered. It is important to only provide the level if pain relief recommended by the veterinarian and consultation must take place before any alterations.

Farriery treatment will involve trimming the hoof in accordance with the radiographic findings. Type one founder will involve addressing a distortion in the toe whilst maintaining sole depth under the pedal bone. Type 2 founder will have an excess of heel that will require lowering carefully ensuring the deep digital flexor tendon doesn't become strained in the process. Trimming from the widest part of the hoof back and engaging the frog with the ground can help achieve this. The dorsal wall should be dressed to reduce flares and distortion where possible but it also important to maintain the structural strength of the hoof wall. Due to the tenderness of the feet, hoof boots may be required post trim for walking across firm surfaces. The addition of a soft deformable pad in the boot will enhance comfort further.

When there is a significant amount of pedal bone rotation and sinkage, then the use of clogs and casts can help to rehabilitate the feet (Fig. 9.13). The author has had many successes using this method over many years. This is due to the ability to place the clog in relation to the position of the pedal bone and reduce leverage to the coffin joint. These can also be applied with screws through predrilled pilot holes, eliminating the need for nailing which would not be possible when the horse is very lame. An anti fungal clay is applied to the sole and frog to help keep the areas healthy whilst there is no access to clean. A soft setting impression material is applied in the rear half of the hoof only as loading the front half with packing can result in further lameness from direct ground pressure towards the tip of the rotated pedal bone. The impression material moulds to the shape of the sole and frog before setting as a complete unit.

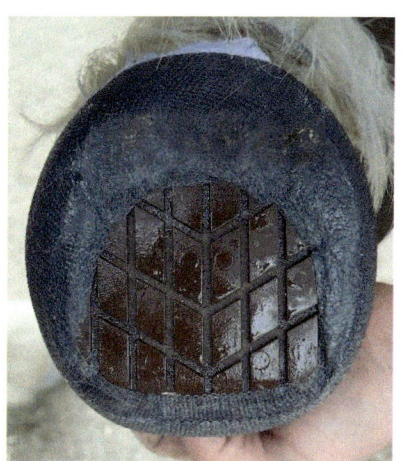

Fig 9.13 Applied clog using screws and cast.

A cast is then applied to the hoof wall and heel bulbs (which are protected rubbing by the cast material by a layer of impression material). The purpose of the cast is to reduce tensile forces on the hoof wall by up to 40%. This also helps to reduce the chances of the hoof distorting over time (Fig. 9.14). Using the biomechanics of the applied clog, over time there is often a reduction in the descent of the pedal bone, a reduction in the rotation of the pedal bone and an increased sole depth (Fig. 9.15 and 9.16). Over time, further trims can result in a normal hoof pastern axis and a healthy strong hoof that can then return to nailed shoes or go barefoot.

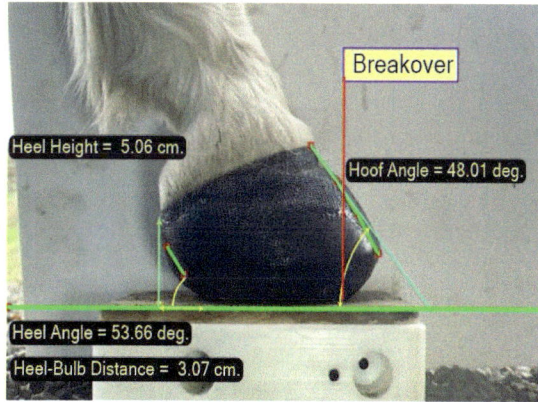

Fig 9.14 Finished clog application with the breakover positioned at the leading edge of the pedal bone.

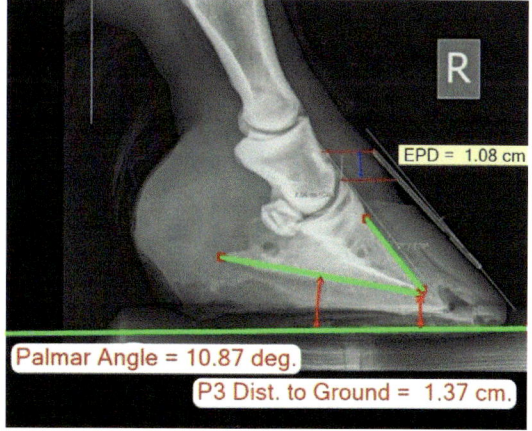

Fig. 9.15 A latero-medio projection showing the position of the pedal bone and sole depth.

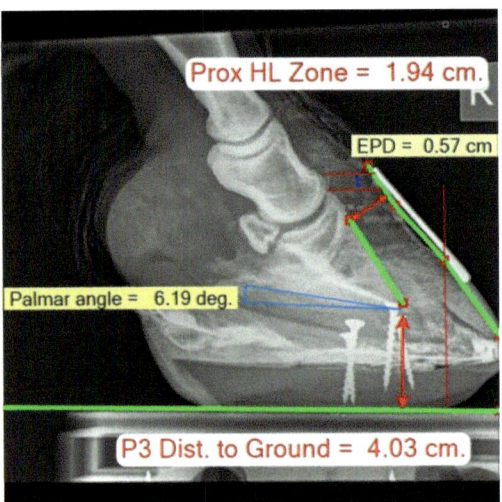

Fig. 9.16 Six weeks after a clog was applied, the pedal bone rotation and descent had reduced along with an increased sole depth.

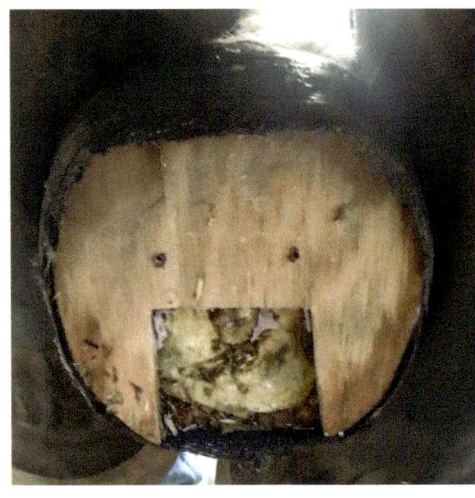

Fig. 9.17 A plywood base with a square cut out to treat the seroma.

There can be cases where access to the sole is required to treat a seroma which is an infection that occurs from the pedal bone rotating into the live sole creating a pressure pocket. The seroma is relived by removing sole with a hoof knife to the pressure pocket following radiography to determine the exact location. These cases require a removable clog and that is achieved by applying a 10mm plywood base with an area cut out in the region of the seroma (Fig. 9.17). This is applied in the same way as a standard clog before the original clog is attached to the plywood base with two screws no longer than the depth of the complete height of both materials combined (Fig. 9.18). This system allows for an easy daily dressing change whilst still maintaining the biomechanics of the clog.

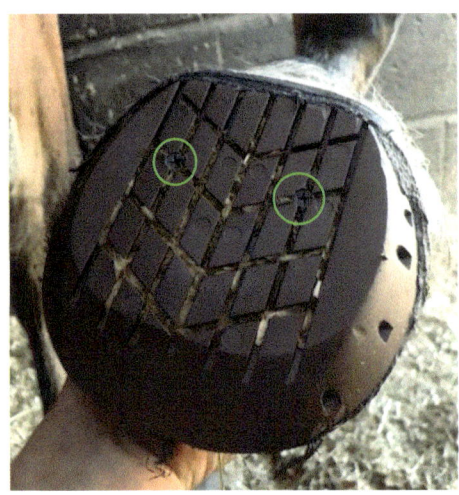

Fig 9.18 Two screws (green circles) hold the plastic clog in position on the plywood base. Cast material acts as a cup to hold the clog in place at the rear of the hoof.

When choosing a nailed shoe option in the recovering laminitic, it is often a good idea to replicate the leverage reduction design of the clog as a transition out of them.

Other options for laminitic horses include glue on thermoplastic heart bar shoes, the author has had some success with these when applied to small ponies (Fig. 9.19). The traditional heart bar shoe combined with pads and impression material can be a good option for mild cases that can accept nailing. These can also be used for horses making a transition out of clogs or to maintain cases long term that require extra protection on the surfaces they work (Fig. 9.20).

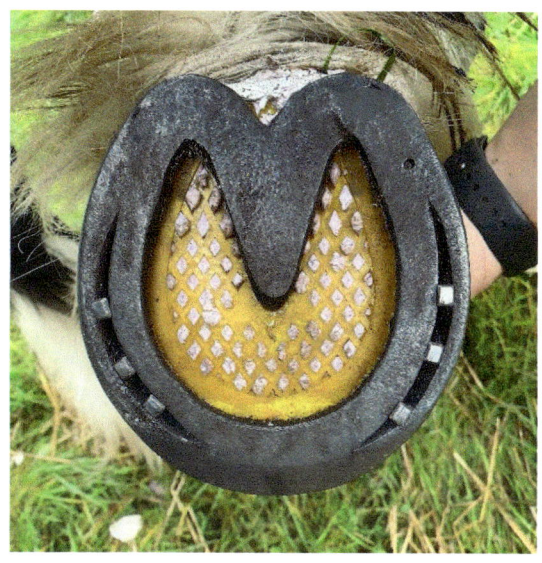

Fig. 9.20 Heart bar shoe made for a recovering laminitic combined with a mesh soe pad and soft setting impression material.

Prognosis

This is variable depending on the comfort of the horse and radiographic findings. If both are poor, then the prognosis is not favourable but if there is considerable improvement in either then a full recovery is possible. There will be a significant change in the horse's management required for long term recovery. Often these horses will struggle to heal in the same environment that made them sick, an overhaul in the diet and workload will often be required to prevent repeat laminitic events.

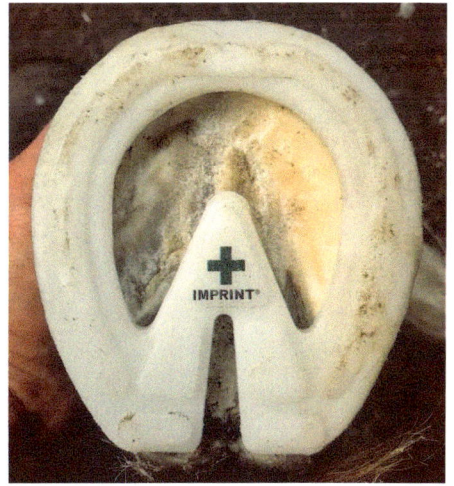

Fig. 9.19 A thermoplastic heart bar shoe glued to the hoof of a laminitic pony.

Coffin joint arthritis

Coffin joint arthritis is also known as degenerative joint disease and effects the joint surfaces most notably at the dorsal margin. There is a progressive degradation of the articular cartilage with periostitis (periosteum inflammation), and exostosis (new bone development) found around the joint margins.

There is a chronic thickening of the synovial membrane that changes the composition of the synovial fluid produced. The articular cartilage gradually thins out as the condition progresses. Lameness can range from mild to severe and horses will struggle particularly when turning and will appear to be short striding when trotted up in a straight line.

Diagnosis

Coffin joint arthritis can be diagnosed using nerve blocks and radiography. A coffin joint block will result in lameness being improved before DP and LM radiography confirming the findings. The arthritis can be categorised into articular (clouding effecting the joint surface) and non articular (clouding on the distal extremity of the pastern bone). An MRI may be performed if any of the surrounding soft tissue structures are suspected to be damaged.

Causes

- Coffin joint arthritis is caused by repeated concussion often as a result of poor conformation.
- Direct trauma from an accident can also lead to a degradation of cartilage.
- Overgrown feet leading to a closure of the dorsal aspect of the coffin joint surface resulting in a breakdown of the articular cartilage.

Treatment

The alignment of the digital bone column should be assessed using radiography and trimmed accordingly to ensure there is no leverage acting on the extensor process of the pedal bone. Quite often the pedal bone will have a low palmar angle resulting in an upward rotation of the dorso-proximal aspect of the pedal bone. This can then result in a "rubbing" of the articular cartilage and therefore allowing the pathology to degenerate. If required, shoeing options can include the use of frog support pads to help with creating alignment along with leverage reduction style shoes (shoes with the edges bevelled off) to help with turning or being worked on a circle. Veterinary treatment can involve the use of injections into the joint using medications such as steroids or polyacrylamide hydrogels such as Arthramid ®. These integrate into the synovial membrane, stabilise the joint capsule and increase elasticity.

Prognosis

Early intervention is key to a successful outcome as the more damage sustained to the joint surface, the more restricted range of motion the joint will have.

Pedal bone fracture

A pedal bone fracture is a split or avulsion to the pedal bone as the result of trauma. There are several classifications of fracture in relation to the location, these are:

Type 1 (Wing fracture) – This is when a piece of the pedal bone is broken away at either the medial or lateral aspect.

Type 2 (Articular fracture) – This is when the fracture extends and involves the joint surfaces of the coffin joint.

Type 3 (Mid sagittal) – This is when the fracture occurs at the front of the pedal bone at the centre, creating an equal division.

Type 4 (Extensor process fracture) – a small fracture at the top of the pedal bone leaving a piece of floating bone just above the coffin joint, this is sometimes referred to as pyramidal disease.

Type 5 (Effusion of the coffin joint) – A fracture of the coffin bone involving the joint that has led to joint effusion.

Type 6 (commuted fracture) – A series of minor fractures along the base of the coffin bone leading to demineralisation of the coffin bone.

Type 7 (foal fracture) – Similar to type 6 fractures although they occur to the rear of the pedal bone and is specific to foals.

Diagnosis

Pedal bone fractures are diagnosed using radiography to determine the location and severity (Fig. 9.20). MRI scans can be performed too if it is considered soft tissue may have been severely damaged (Heer at al. 2020)

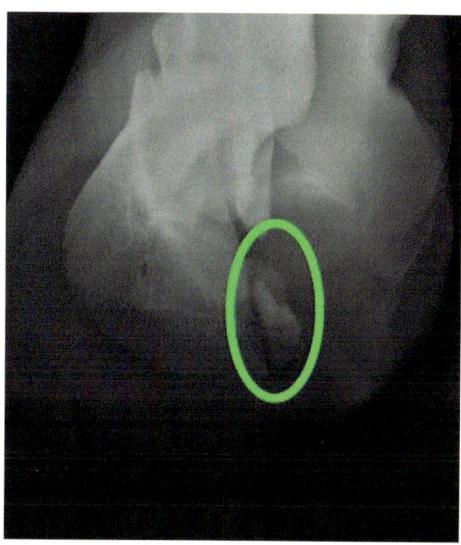

Fig. 9.20 A wing fracture of the coffin bone highlighted in the green circle.

Treatment

Box rest is often required to prevent movement delaying the recovery process. Farriery treatment can involve the use of a bar shoe with multiple clips to completely stabilise the hoof, but care must be taken to apply as few nails as possible during the early stages of recovery (Kidd, 2011).

Glue on shoes with a large cuff could also be considered if nailing is an issue along with pads and packing. The use of a hoof cast is what the author considers to be the most effective for stabilising the hoof with a simple and efficient application that requires no nailing (Fig. 9.21 and 9.22). This should be kept on for 6 weeks

Conditions of the Pedal Bone and Coffin Joint

before a fresh set of radiographs to monitor the progress of recovery.

Prognosis

The prognosis for most fractures is good with many horses returning to full work with little evidence of the injury.

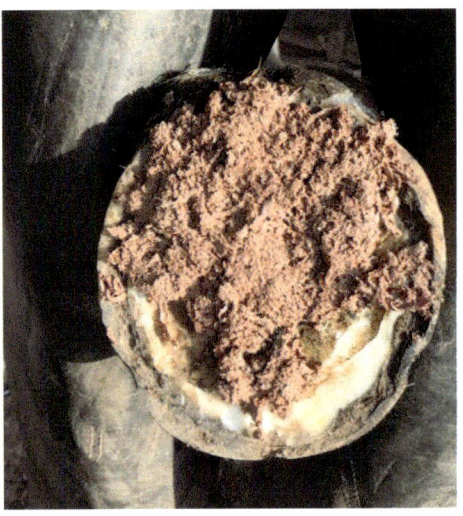

Fig. 9.21 Hoof packing comprised of shreds of leather soaking in anti-bacterial solution.

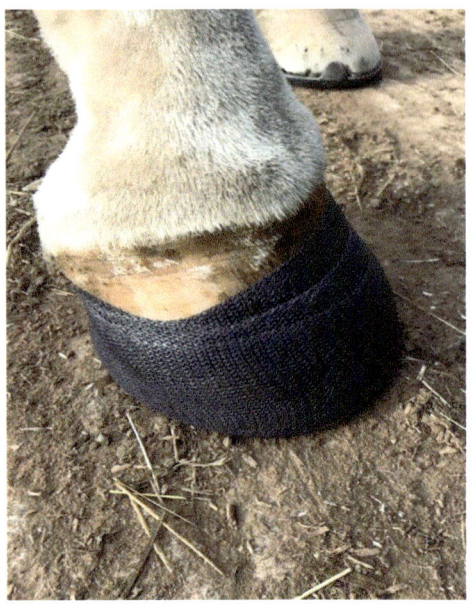

Fig. 9.22 A hoof cast applied to a hoof with a fractured pedal bone.

Sidebone

Sidebone refers to an ossification of the collateral cartilages of the hoof which can happen either on one side (unilateral) or both sides (bilateral) of the pedal bone (Fig. 9.23). These cartilages are attached to the proximal borders of the palmar processes of the coffin bone and are palpable to hand due to extending above the coronary band.

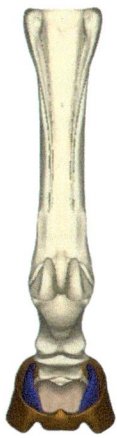

Fig. 9.23 Location of the dorso collateral cartilages of the hoof (purple). *

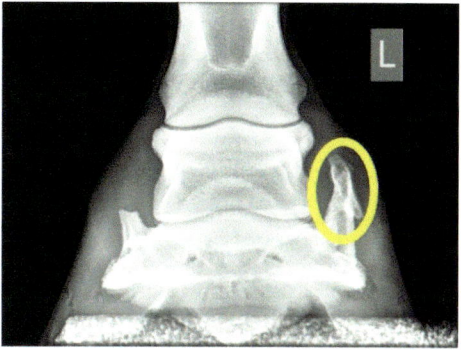

Fig. 9.24 A radiograph showing an area of ossification at the dorso collateral cartilage. This is defined as unilateral sidebone.

The cartilages are composed of hyaline and fibrous tissue with their main function to act as part of the anti-concussive mechanism of the hoof along with aiding circulation due to the coronary venous plexus vessels passing through the cartilage.

Diagnosis

Lameness is often present during the time the cartilage is forming to bone and can subside once full ossification has taken place. There can sometimes be two areas of ossification taking place and careful assessment must take place to not confuse this with a sidebone fracture which carries a worse prognosis (Cullimore and Booth, 2010).

Sidebone is diagnosed using radiography with a large spur seen branching out from the pedal bone (Fig. 9.24).

The hoof can sometimes become medio-lateral unbalanced as the hoof compensates for the pain felt during weight bearing. There can also be excessive shoe wear to the side of the hoof that is suffering from new bone formation, and it is good practice to mimic this in any new shoe applied along with a removal of any traction applications such as tungsten pins to allow for a smooth slide when the hoof contacts the ground as opposed to a sharp brake.

Navicular syndrome

Navicular syndrome refers to pain experienced at the rear half of the front hooves involving the navicular bone and/or its surrounding structures. There is a gradual shortening of the horse's stride with most displaying a toe first hoof landing along with a tendency to trip or stumble. Lameness will increase when worked on a hard surface or in a circle.

The lameness can be either unilateral (one hoof) or bilateral (both feet). Cases of unilateral lameness tend to have feet that develop in dissimilar size and shape with the lame hoof becoming smaller and more contracted due to reluctance to bear weight upon it (Eggleston et al. 2020). Cases of bilateral lameness tend to develop feet with low weak and contracted heels due to a reluctance to load the rear third of the hoof and therefore a toe first, secondary heel compression loading pattern is established.

The most common structures effected with navicular syndrome include:

- Navicular bone – changes in density or to the articular surface.
- Distal impar ligament – The ligament between the navicular and coffin bone can become inflamed.
- Deep digital flexor tendon – This passes over the navicular bone before attaching to the semi lunar line of the pedal bone (Fig. 9.25). This can suffer from tears, strains or lesions to the navicular bone.
- Navicular bursa – A small fluid filled structure that acts a cushion where the deep digital flexor tendon passes over the bone. This can suffer from inflammation as a consequence of repeated concussion.

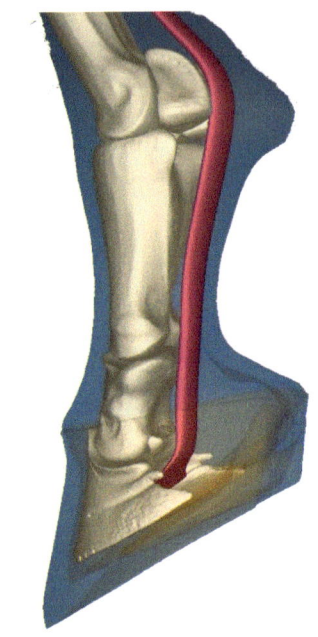

Fig. 9.25 The deep digital flexor tendon passing over the navicular bone before a final wide insertion onto the semi lunar line of the distal phalanx. *

There are two theories as to why the pain develops in the rear of the hoof:

Vascular compromise – Low oxygen levels in the tissues and bone are caused by blood clots. The bone is then likely to degenerate as a result of a lack of oxygen and arterial occlusion.

Biomechanical theory – Abnormal forces arise from excessive loading as a result of poor conformation or horses with mismatched front feet. These excessive forces result in a remodelling of the navicular bone.

Diagnosis

A palmar digital nerve block will help to establish if lameness is present in the rear of the hoof. A navicular bursa block can also be used to further establish the localised area of pain. Navicular syndrome can be diagnosed with radiography if bone damage is involved with views of the lateromedial, dorsoproximal-palmarodistal, dorsoproximal-palmarodistal oblique and palmaroproximal-palmarodistal oblique projections taken to give multiple views of the navicular bone (Fig. 9.26).

If navicular syndrome is present, there will be an increase in the number of foraminae (holes) in the navicular bone with increased bone density between these foraminae (Komosa et al. 2018). This is due to an increase of blood vessels attempting to pass through the bone and help nourish the bone.

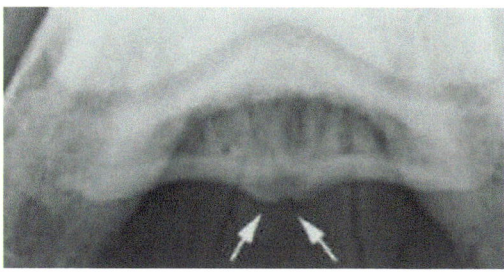

Fig. 9.26 Palmaroproximal palmarodistal oblique radiograph showing several large lucent zones on the navicular bone as well as a large radiolucent defect in the flexor cortex at the sagittal ridge (white arrows).

Quite often, it is desirable to obtain an MRI of the hoof to assess damage to the surrounding soft tissue structures of the navicular bone as radiography will only account of half of the diagnostics (Fig 9.27). The increased signal densities highlight areas of pain and inflammation.

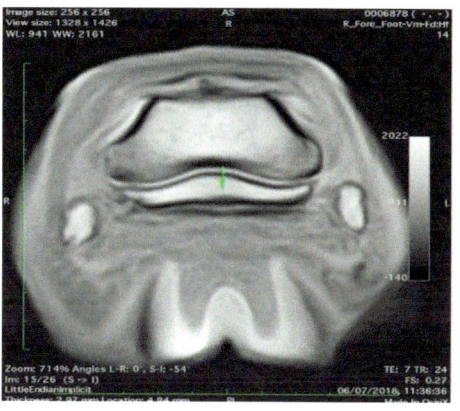

Fig. 9.27 MRI showing a moderate signal increase in the region of the navicular bursa.

Causes

- Poor conformation with broken back or broken forward hoof pastern axis resulting in an excessive overdevelopment or underdevelopment of the rear of the hoof and as a consequence, excessive force being placed upon the navicular bone and associated structures.
- Excessive work on hard surfaces creating repetitive concussion.
- Long or overdue feet creating a reduction in the tendinous surface of the navicular bone as the deep digital flexor tendon passes over it. This is due to the navicular bone changing in the

Conditions of the Pedal Bone and Coffin Joint

angle it makes with the ground surface.

Treatment

Farriery treatment will revolve around the target of reducing concussion the rear of the hoof and creating alignment of the bone column. There are some horses that respond well to going barefoot with a change in diet and management of the horse (Fig. 9.28).

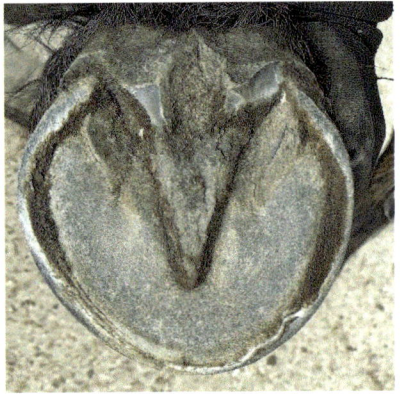

Fig. 9.28 A horse with navicular syndrome that has responded well to barefoot rehabilitation. Note the development of the rear of the hoof and expanded heels.

However, there are some where their environment doesn't allow for this, and corrective shoes are required. A correct and full diagnosis is essential for choosing the style of shoe to apply. A short term application of a roller motion egg bar shoe with the edges bevelled off to reduce hoof leverage (Fig. 9.29 and 9.30).

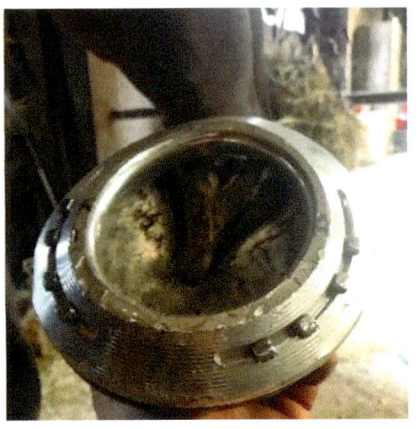

Fig. 9.29 Aluminium roller motion egg bar shoe helping to provide smooth landing and breakover to the hoof.

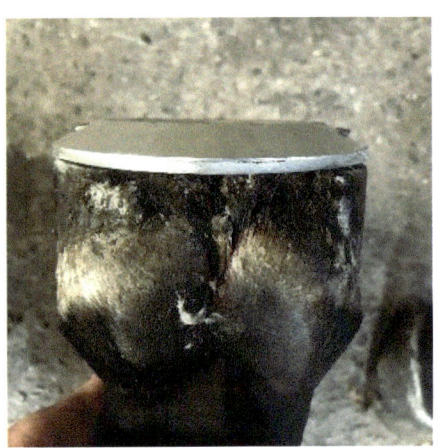

Fig 9.30 The heel bar provides load sharing across the rear of the hoof.

There are some horses that will benefit from a frog support pad to help adjust the palmar angle of the pedal bone and the tendinous surface angle of the navicular bone (Fig. 9.31).

Conditions of the Pedal Bone and Coffin Joint

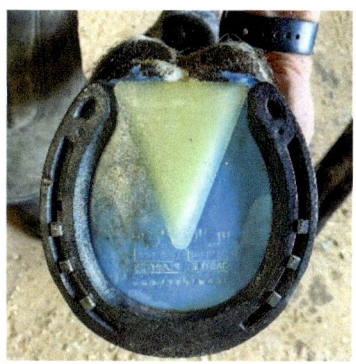

Fig. 9.31 A synthetic frog support pad combined with soft setting impression material providing protection to an area exposed to excessive concussion.

Variations of these can include heel pads which are applied with a half shoe to offer barefoot function of the rear of the hoof whilst also offering shod protection at the same time (Fig. 9.32).

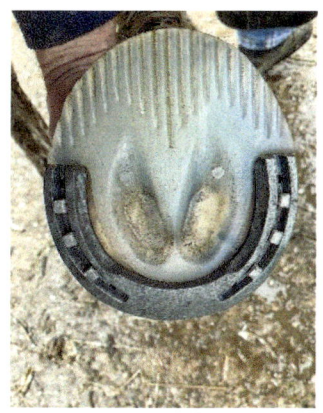

Fig. 9.32 A heel pad shoe that can be lifted at the rear half to clean out the frog.

Steel frog supports are usually the last resort if all other options have been exhausted (Fig. 9.33). This is due to the risk of increasing concussion to the navicular structures, however, there have been cases that have responded well to stability at the rear of the hoof using this method particularly if combined with a soft setting hoof packing.

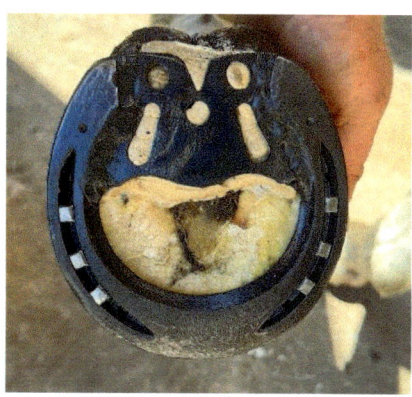

Fig. 9.33 A wide plate frog support welded in a shoe with soft setting hoof packing.

Prognosis

The prognosis is often guarded with navicular syndrome depending on the level of damage sustained during the initial onset. Constant care and management will be required in the long term to prevent further degradation.

Pedal osteitis

Pedaloseitis is an inflammation around the pedal bone that eventually leads to a demineralisation of the peripheral border of the bone. This can occur as a result of repeated concussion from hard surfaces or flat thin soles being unable to provide adequate protection to the underlying sensitive structures. These horses will struggle perform well on hard ground and will require sole protection either in the form of a pad or protective hoof boot to prevent further deterioration of the pedal bone.

Septic Pedal osteitis

This occurs as result of infection, puncture wound or chronic laminitis (Carlson, 2022). The demineralisation of the pedal bone is similar to non septic cases but often lameness is more severe (Fig. 9.34). If there is an infected pedal bone present, then surgery will be required to remove the necrotic area. A hospital plate is then required to allow for daily access and treatment of the infected area. The chances of returning to full work are low but there are cases that can be managed well with protective sole pads.

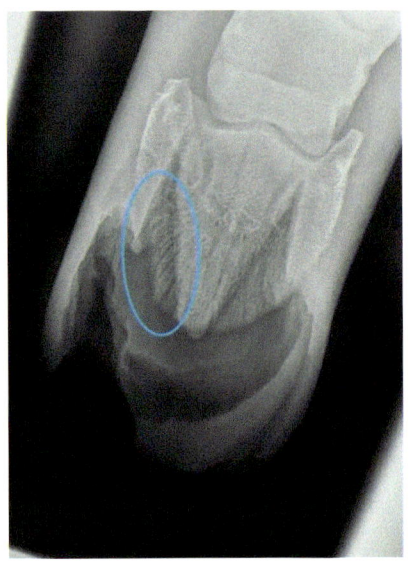

Fig. 9.34 An example of demineralisation of the coffin bone as a result of a deep hoof abscess.

References

Butler, D & Butler, J. (2004) '*The Principles of Horseshoeing (P3)*', Doug Butler Enterprises: Colorado, USA.

Carlson, N. (2022). Foreign Body Penetration of the Hoof. In *Comparative Veterinary Anatomy* (pp. 918-924). Academic Press.

Colles, C., Ware, R., & Hayes, J. (2022) '*Principles of Farriery*' The Crowood Press: Marlborough

Cullimore, A., & Booth, T. (2010) 'Clinical aspects of the equine foot Part 6: The collateral cartilages' *UK Vet Companion Animal*, Vol. 15, No.8, pp 9-12.

Eggleston, R. B., Baxter, G. M., Belknap, J., Parks, A., Dern, K., Watts, A. E., & Bertone, A. L. (2020) 'Lameness of the distal limb: navicular region/palmar foot' *Adams and Stashak's Lameness in Horses*, pp 439-595.

Heer, C., Fürst, A. E., Del Chicca, F., & Jackson, M. A. (2020) 'Comparison of 3D-assisted surgery and conservative methods for treatment of type III fractures of the distal phalanx in horses' *Equine Veterinary Education*, Vol. 32, pp 42-51.

Johnson, P. J., Wiedmeyer, C. E., LaCarrubba, A., Ganjam, V. S., & Messer, N. T. (2010) 'Laminitis and the equine metabolic syndrome' *Veterinary Clinics: Equine Practice*, Vol. 26, No.2 pp 239-255.

Kidd, J. (2011) 'Pedal bone fractures', *Equine Veterinary Education*, vol. 23, pp 314-323.

Komosa, M., Włodarek, J., Dzierzęcka, M., Nienartowicz-Zdrojewska, A., & Tołkacz, M. (2018) 'Comparison of pathological lesions in navicular bone (os sesamoideum distale) and analysis of remodelling capacity' *Polish Journal of Veterinary Sciences*, Vol. 21, No.1, pp 13-27.

Pollitt, C. C. (2004) 'Equine laminitis', *Clinical Techniques in equine practice*, Vol. 3, No.1, pp 34-44.

Van Eps, A., Collins, S. N., & Pollitt, C. C. (2010) 'Supporting limb laminitis' *Veterinary Clinics: Equine Practice*, Vol. 26, No.2 pp 287-302.

* Images adapted with kind permission from Effigos AG. Hoof Explorer

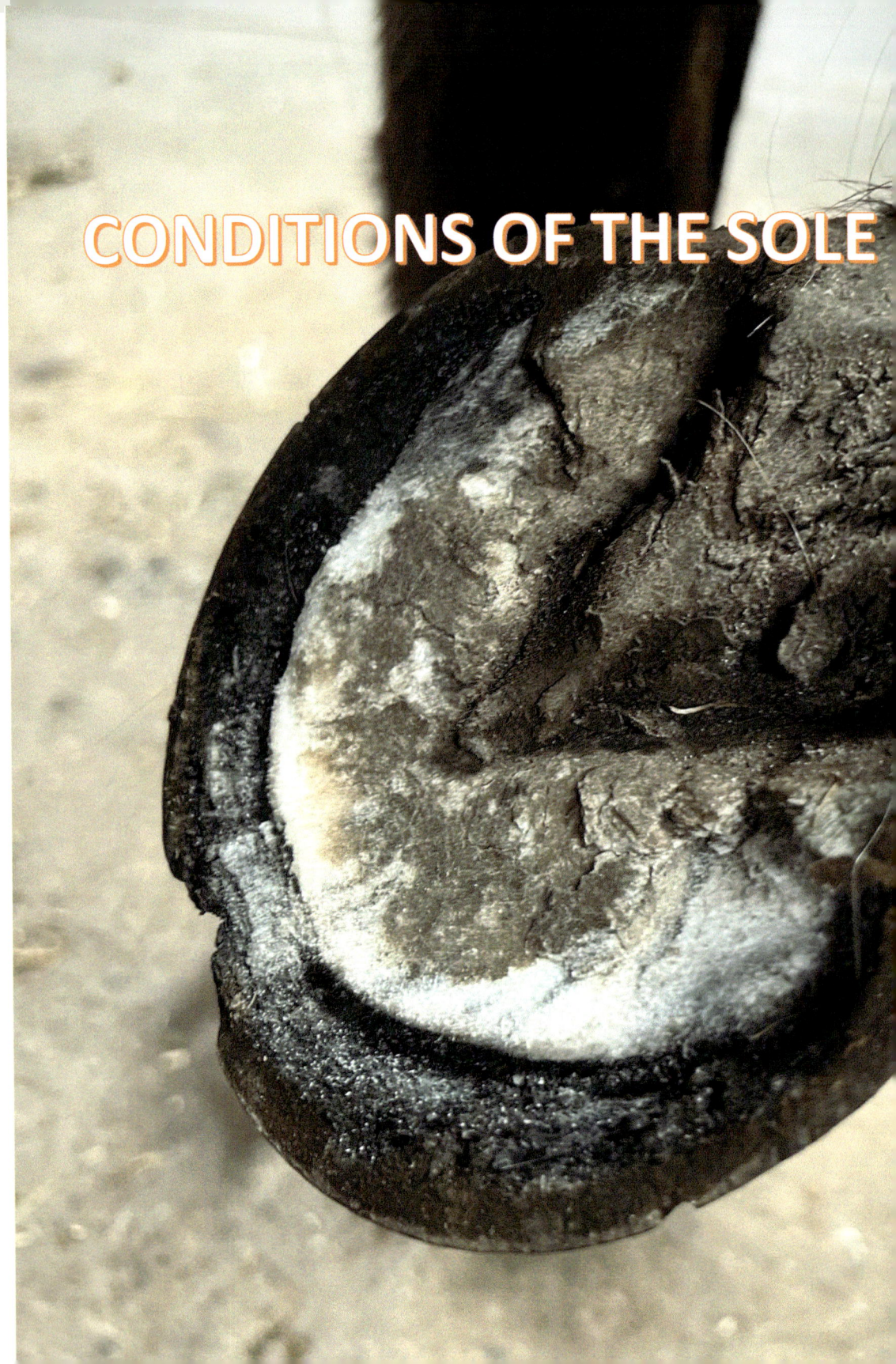

CONDITIONS OF THE SOLE

Chapter 10 - Conditions of the sole

Introduction

The sole surface of the hoof allows the horse to feel the ground and allow for grip during locomotion. The outer hoof wall is attached to the sole by the white line and laminae. The frog is found in the centre of the hoof being widest at the rear portion before tapering to a point as it travels towards the front third of the hoof (Fig. 10.1).

The horn of the sole is produced at the solar corium below the pedal bone and is said to have a moisture content of around 33% (Fig. 10.2). The arch of the sole relates to how concave the sole shape is, some low heeled feet have a flat sole arch and in some cases of laminitis, the sole becomes convex as a result of the pedal bone sinking into the horny sole.

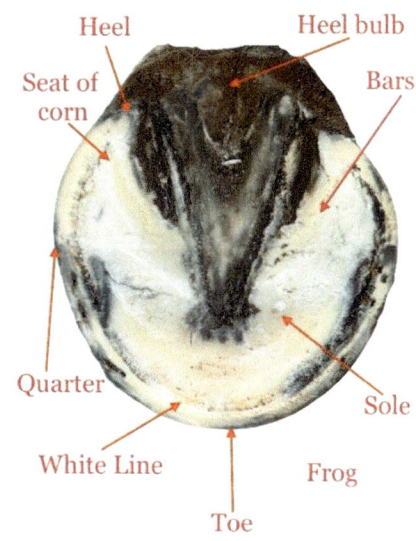

Fig. 10.1 References points of the sole.

Conditions of the sole

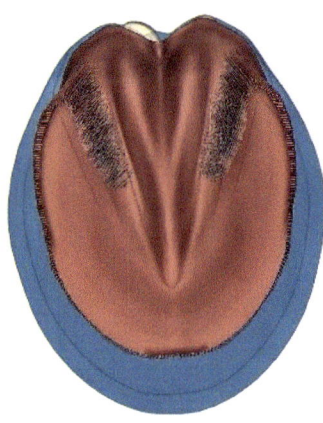

Fig. 10.2 The solar corium that creates sole horn to protect the internal structures of the hoof. *

Retracted soles

There are many terms that can be used to describe a sole that has drawn inwards but the most common is "retracted sole". This is when the sole assumes a deep concavity drawn upwards towards the pedal bone (Fig. 10.3). This usually occurs when spring arrives and if there is a sudden change in weather, the sole dries out quickly and if mud has etched away at the layers of sole horn it loses its rigidity. This can also occur in environments that many genetic horses are not adapted to such as high rainfall areas, subsequently there is invasion by opportunistic pathogens that cause manifestations such as retracted soles, thrush or mud fever (Holzhauer et al. 2017).

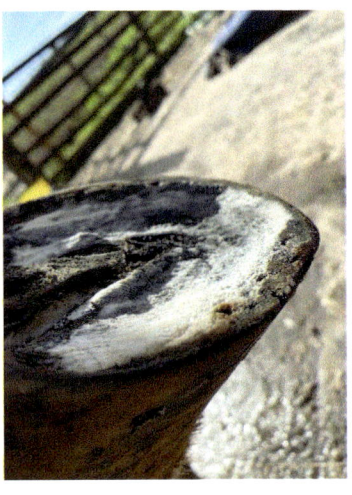

Fig. 10.3 A sole on an ex racehorse that has become drawn upwards creating a deep concavity of sole that is of little thickness.

This can lead to a deception that there is a lot of hoof to trim off but in reality, there will be far less, and care should be taken before deciding to remove any sole.

Treatment

Most cases return to their original state over a course of two months but if there is lameness present it could be due to bruising of the sole. Protective hoof boots or pads under shoes can be used to allow the sole to regenerate and protect against hard ground. A spray solution of iodine can help to draw out moisture and help to harden the sole.

Sole bruise

Sole bruises appear as red specks on the solear surface of the hoof. Blood vessels in the sensitive structures rupture due to trauma and stain the horny sole (Fig. 10.4). Sole bruises occur from direct trauma to the hoof or repetitive concussion over a long period of time. They can occur in the shod and unshod hoof but horses with a flatter sole are more prone due to their inability to resist hard ground concussion (Bowe, 2015).

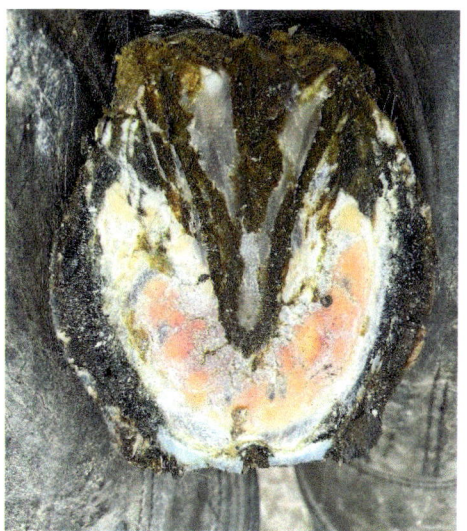

Fig. 10.4 A sole bruise evident by the red pigmentation as a result of inflammation.

If lameness is present, it would be best practice to contact a veterinarian in case any pain relief is required. It may take a while for discolouration of the sole to appear and usually appears once lameness has been abolished. Certain anti inflammatory hoof packers under pads can be beneficial due to containing Absorbine which helps to draw out bruising, but care must be taken however to not overload an area already in a pain.

Corns

Corns occur at the junction of the bars of the hoof and the white line towards the heel area. They are effectively an area of bruising and trauma due to repetitive concussion (Fig. 10..5). Corns are commonly associated with low weak heels and horses that have had their shoes on for too long. Barefoot horses do not tend to develop corns and whilst corns can develop in hind feet, they are rarely seen.

Lameness can vary from mild to severe with infected corns taking longer to recover.

Conditions of the sole

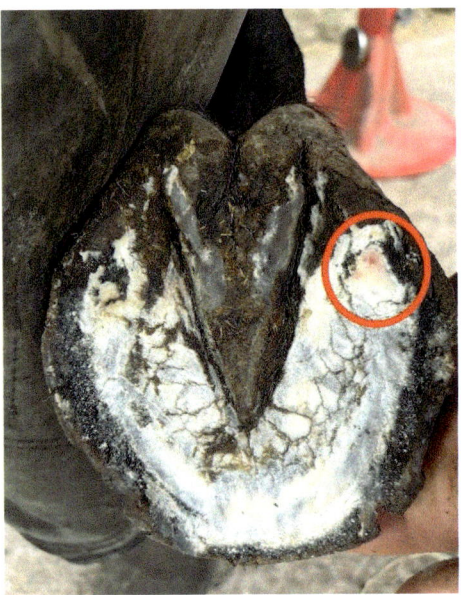

Fig. 10.5 A corn highlighted by the red circle showing a red tinge to the seat of corn.

Over a period of time concussive forces will increase on the low weak heels and create internal bruising. When the hoof is trimmed, a circular red area will appear.

Treatment

A corn will require the hoof to remain without a shoe and daily hot saltwater bathing to help draw out bruising. Once the horse has started to show signs of improvement, then shoes can be reapplied quite often, the application of a frog support in either a pad or heart bar shoe will help to reduce loading forces off the heels and utilise the frog as a load share. A wide webbed shoe along with a shorter shoeing cycle can also be used for successful treatment.

Suppurating corn

A suppurating corn is a corn that has gone septic and resulted in infection. Treatment of this will involve poulticing for a week or until the infection is clear and dried up.

Hoof puncture

Hoof punctures occur as a result of stepping on a sharp object and a laceration occurs to the solear aspect of the hoof (Fig. 10.6). This can result in bleeding and non weight bearing lameness (Fig. 10.7). If there is a foreign object lodged within the sole, it is strongly advised to obtain a radiograph first to monitor the depth of penetration and to determine if any surgery is then required (O'Neill & O'Meara, 2010).

Conditions of the sole

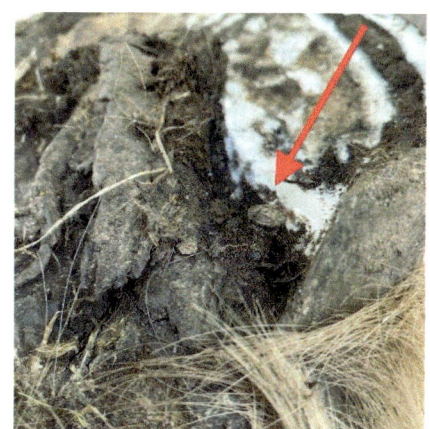

Fig. 10.6 A fencing nail penetrating the rear of the frog.

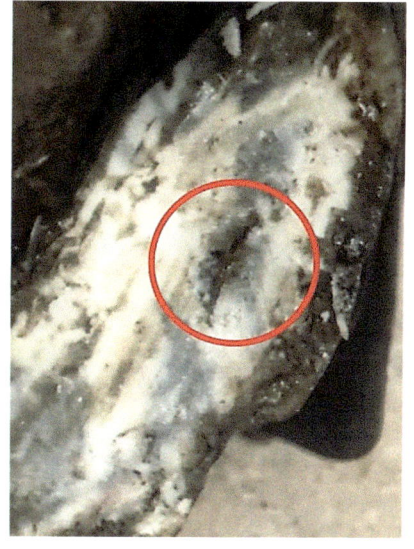

Fig. 10.7 The red circle indicating a puncture site to the sole of the hoof.

Underrun sole

An underrun sole develops because of an infection that then creates a cavity as the bacteria spreads (Fig. 10.8). Lameness has usually become resolved as the initial infection has either been treated or went unnoticed (Barr, 2019). In order to prevent any further infection, applying iodine in a spray bottle to the area can help eliminate remaining bacteria. There may be some cases where the sole remains tender and these benefit from application of pads with shreds of leather packing that are soaked in anti septic solution. This is placed underneath the pads for at least one shoeing cycle whilst the sole regenerates (Redding & O'Grady, 2012).

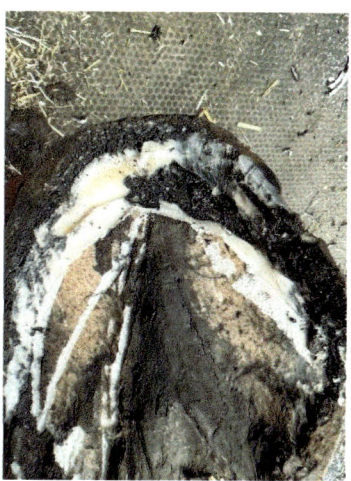

Fig. 10.8 An example of a black cavity full of bacteria in an underrun sole.

References

Barr, E. (2019) 'Foot abscessation in horses' *The Veterinary Record*, Vol. *184, No*.8, pp 249-259.

Baxter, G. M. (Ed.). (2020). *Adams and Stashak's lameness in horses.* John Wiley & Sons: New Jersey, USA.

Bowe, A. (2015) 'MSM and healthy hooves', *Horses and people*, Vol. 6, pp 53-59.

Holzhauer, M., Bremer, R., Santman-Berends, I., Smink, O., Janssens, I., & Back, W. (2017) 'Cross-sectional study of the prevalence of and risk factors for hoof disorders in horses in The Netherlands' *Preventive veterinary medicine*, Vol. *140*, pp 53-59.

O'Neill, H., & O'Meara, B. (2010) 'Diagnosis and treatment of penetrating injuries of the hoof in horses' *In Practice*, Vol. *32*, No.10, pp 484-490.

Redding, W. R., & O'Grady, S. E. (2012) 'Septic diseases associated with the hoof complex: abscesses, punctures wounds, and infection of the lateral cartilage' *Veterinary Clinics of North America: Equine Practice*, Vol. *28, No*.2, pp 423-440.

* Images adapted with kind permission from Effigos AG. Hoof Explorer

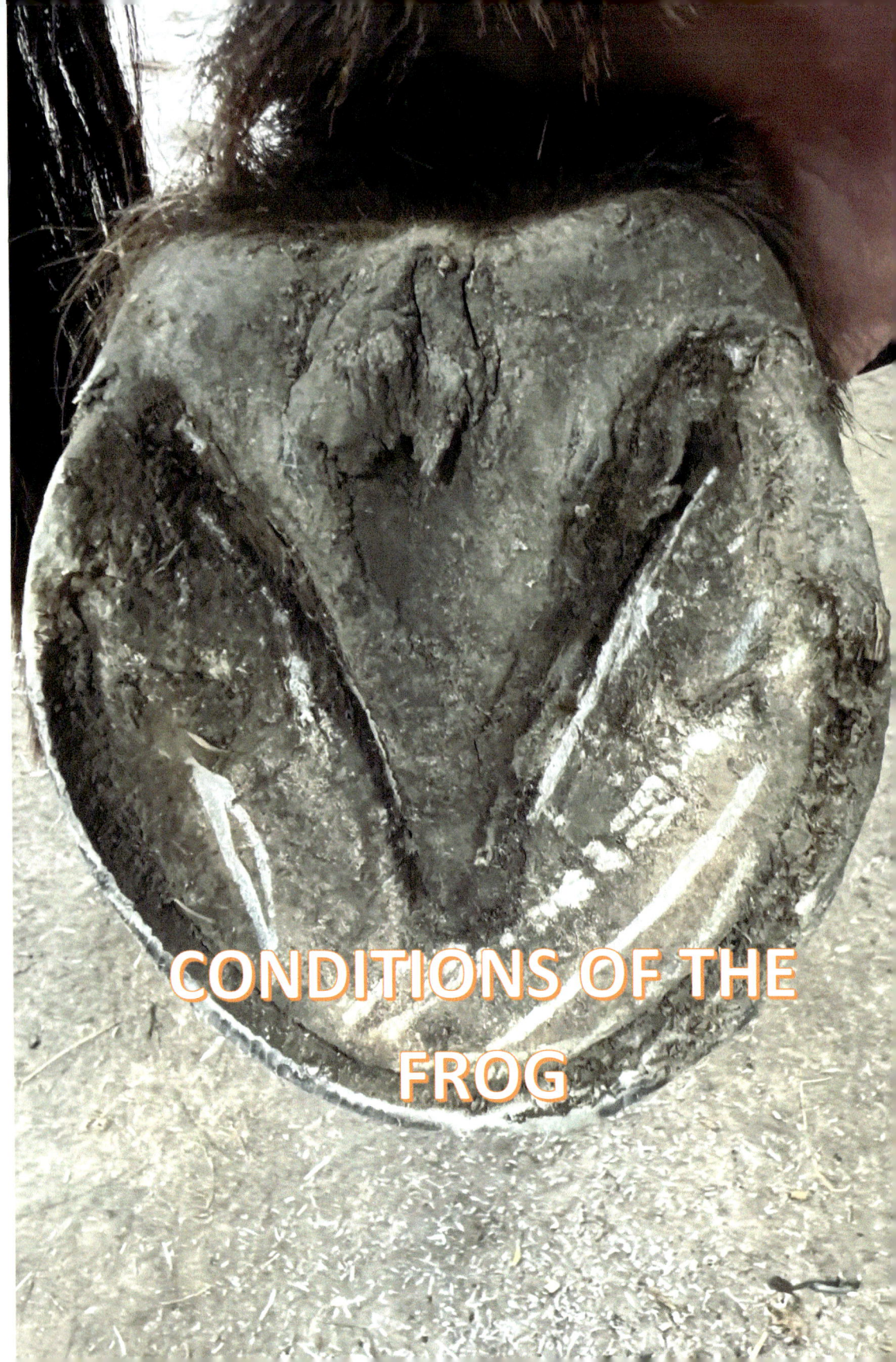

CONDITIONS OF THE FROG

Chapter 11 - Conditions of the Frog

Introduction

The frog is a wedged shape piece of elastic horn occupying the area between the bars of the sole. The grooves on either side of the frog are called the commissures with the groove in the centre of the frog being the central sulcus (Fig 11.1). The frog contains horn tubules that are slightly bent towards the ground surface, sweat glands originating from the digital cushion pass through these tubules from the sensitive frog into the horny frog. The sweat glands that are secreted help the frog to maintain an elastic structure with the frog containing an approximately 50% moisture content (Fig. 11.2).

The function of the frog is to allow expansion of the heels, provide grip for the hoof and act as part of the anti concussive mechanisms of the hoof. The frog is developed at the frog corium and is often characterised in its shape with the amount of contact with the ground (Fig. 11.3).

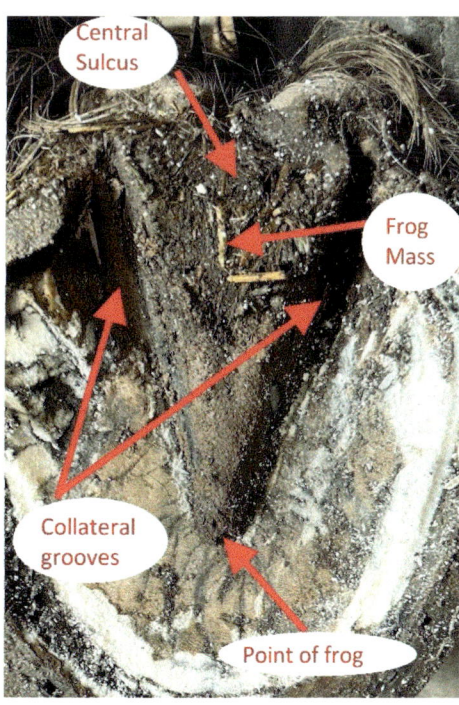

Fig. 11.2 The anatomical reference points of the frog.

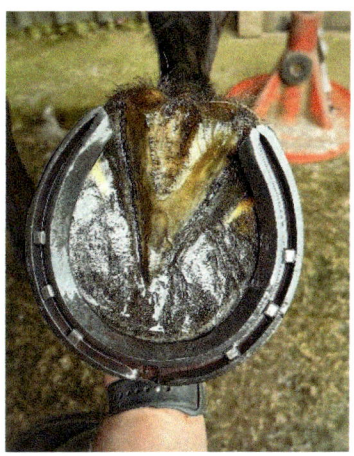

Fig. 11.1 An example of a healthy strong frog.

Conditions of the frog

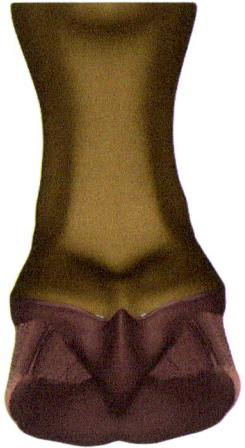

Fig. 11.3 The frog is developed at the frog corium found within the hoof capsule. *

A well functioning frog that has ground contact and engagement during the stance phase is likely to be wider in order to be functional at absorbing concussion. A narrow frog drawn back into the hoof is unlikely to have much ground contact resulting in a loss of function for protecting the internal sensitive structures. The frog will shed in its entirety several times a year. However, due to regular trimming and friction from the ground wearing away the frog horn this is rarely seen and is only observed in horses overdue for trimming.

Management advice for the frog

A simple procedure of daily hoof picking when brought in from the field and/or removed from the stable is advised with the commissures of the frog fully cleaned to prevent dirt and bacteria becoming built up. Ensuring a clean stable with absorbent bedding is advised to help dry out the frogs and allow the hoof to stand on a clean surface.

Whilst there is little that can be done about soil conditions without an extensive overhaul to the turnout area, consider applying a firm surface to where the horses eat their hay. This could be concrete or with mud control mats which will help to reduce the time spent in deep wet going.

Preventative treatment of the frog also has its merits with more success seen with solutions that dry the horn out such as anti fungal hoof clays as opposed to wet solutions due the nature of the anaerobic bacteria thriving on the moisture.

Thrush

Thrush is a bacterial infection of the frog characterised by a black discharge from the frog and an unpleasant odour. The bacteria associated with thrush is known as *Fusobaterium necrophorum* which exists in an anaerobic environment such as dirt or manure (Agne, 2010). If this becomes packed in the hoof, the bacteria will attack the healthy tissue of the frog due to its flexible state, making it easier to penetrate through than the sole.

The infection usually occurs at the central sulcis of the frog resulting in a deep split that can penetrate sensitive tissue (Fig. 11.4). If left untreated, lameness can occur and further damage to healthy tissue will take place. The infection is associated with poor hygiene or ground conditions.

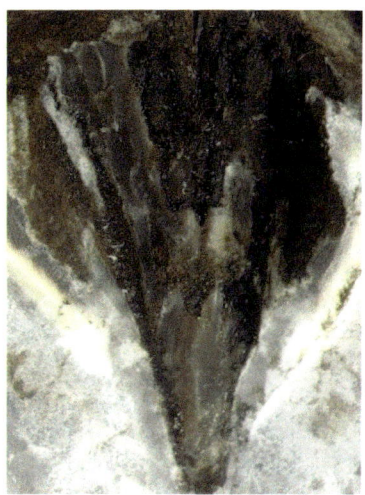

Fig. 11. 4 A thrush infection of the frog resulting in black discharge in the central sulcis.

Rubber matting is also a contributor to infection due to the reduction of bedding applied, the horse stands a lot in their own waste whilst urine is absorbed into the rubber matting making it hard to provide a clean environment as bacteria cannot drain away.

Treatment

The frog should be trimmed by a farrier to safely remove any necrotic or damaged tissue and to reinstate a normal wedge shape as possible. There may be some cases where the frog has atrophied (worn away or become drawn inwards and upwards) and trimming may not be possible due to how sensitive the remaining horn is (Petrov & Dicks, 2013).

Daily hoof picking, particularly those with deep frog clefts will help to reduce the chances of infection. Applying an anti bacterial hoof clay to the central sulcis of the frog will prevent any debris from entering along with helping to regenerate tissue. Antifungal clay will also help to dry out a saturated frog and impregnate natural ingredients and antibacterial properties into the developmental tissues of the frog (Fig. 11.5). Topical antibacterial spray such as oxytetracycline can also be used for treating thrush. Wood pellets act as the perfect bedding for these types of infections due to the fact they can dry out moisture and absorb bacteria.

Consider having the soil in your turnout paddock tested for the minerals and pH levels, the more alkaline the soil, the higher the chance of thrush infection. Where possible, soil treatments can alter the acidity and help to prevent further infections.

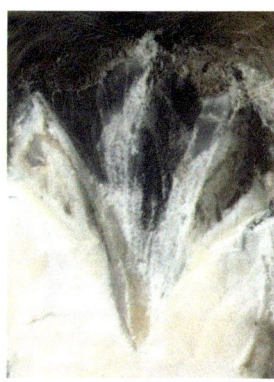

Fig. 11.5 A healthy frog following treatment with no diseased material and an expansion in size due to a strong complete structure.

Conditions of the frog

Canker

Canker is a rare pathology of the frog resulting in diseased material destroying healthy tissue and creating moderate to severe lameness. The condition itself is dissimilar to thrush as the hypertrophy of the frog results in a large mass of diseased growth with the blood supply becoming damaged and irregular (Fig. 11.6).

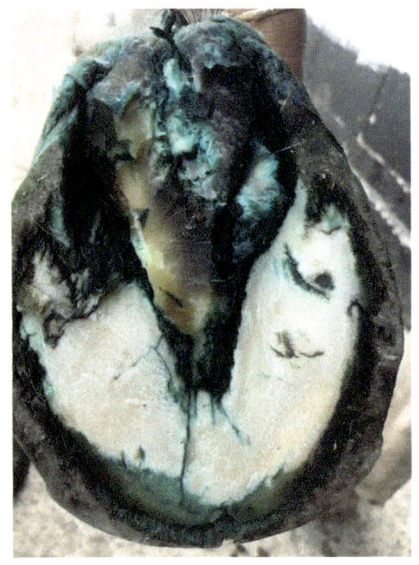

Fig. 11.6 Development of canker at the right hand side of the frog.

The cause is unknown but is considered a hyper reactive response to chronic anaerobic infection. This infection causes benign growths to be produced and there is no demarcation between sensitive and horny frog (Apprich et al. 2017). There will be a large mass of cheese like growth, light in colour with an unpleasant smell, distinctively different from thrush and is comparable with necrotic tissue (Fig. 11.7).

The frog will be sensitive to touch and great care should be taken when picking out the feet prior to treatment.

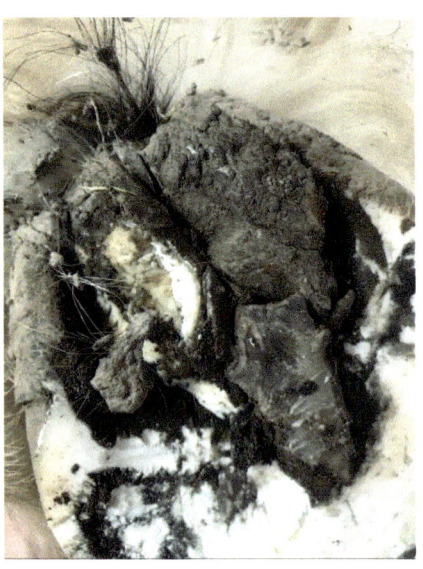

Fig. 11.7 An example of severe canker infection that has invaded the entire frog.

Treatment

The diseased material will be required to be removed under veterinary supervision due to sensitive structures being breached along with a large discharge of blood (Fig. 11.8). A torniquet should be applied to the lower limb to help stem the amount of blood flow and to make it easier to debride back to healthy frog horn (Oosterlinck et al. 2011). Once this is complete, a waterproof dressing should be applied using swabs across the frog with a treatment solution (Fig 11.9 and 11.10).

Conditions of the frog

Maximum pressure should be applied to the frog to help stimulate new growth during recovery. The treatment applications vary and, in some cases, will take trial and error to see success. The most common treatments include potassium permanganate, metronidazole tablets, copper sulphate powder and eucalyptus oil. This is applied directly to the frog with a large swab placed on top before wrapping up the dressing either with vet wrap or under a hospital plate that is bolted to the ground surface of a shoe (Fig 11.11 and 11.12).

The horse will require box rest during recovery to reduce the chances of moisture, dirt and bacteria making their way under the dressing.

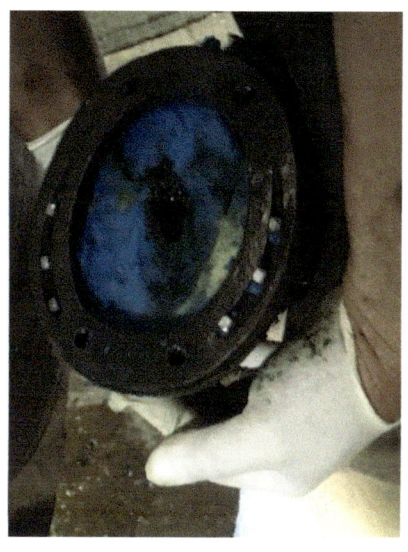

Fig. 11.9 Packing the frog and sole with copper sulphate and vinegar.

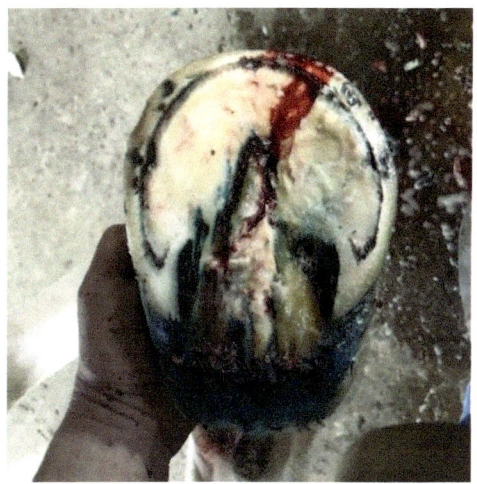

Fig. 11.8 The diseased material removed back to healthy horn.

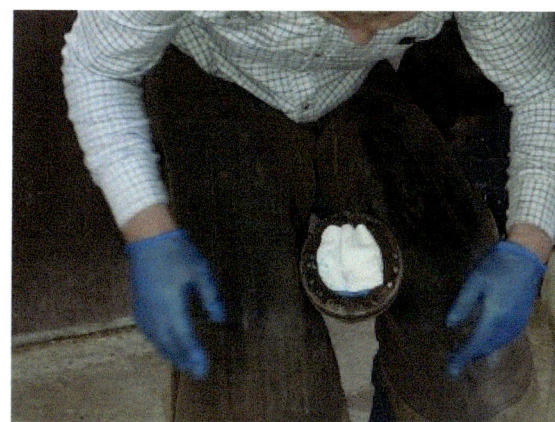

Fig. 11.10 Swabs applied to provide maximum pressure to the frog.

Conditions of the frog

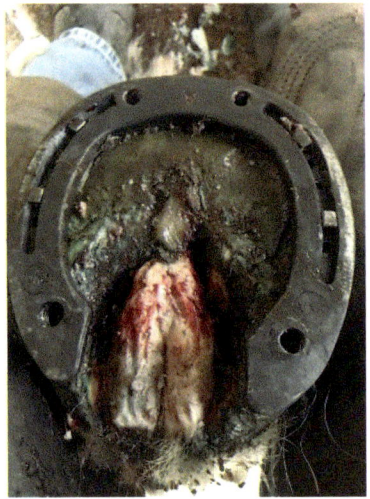

Fig. 11.11 An open heel shoe or a bar shoe can be applied with 10mm holes drilled and threaded for a hospital plate with removable bolts to allow access for treatment.

As the infection recovers it is possible to treat the remainder of infection with daily dressing changes and regular hoof trimming with the aim for the frog to make ground contact so that it redevelops its functional wedge shape (Fig. 11.13). Once the frog is free from canker infestation then turnout can begin along with light work (Fig.11.14).

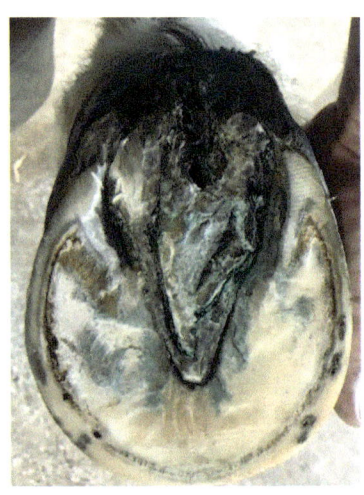

Fig. 11.13 Progress after a month with new healthy horn being generated.

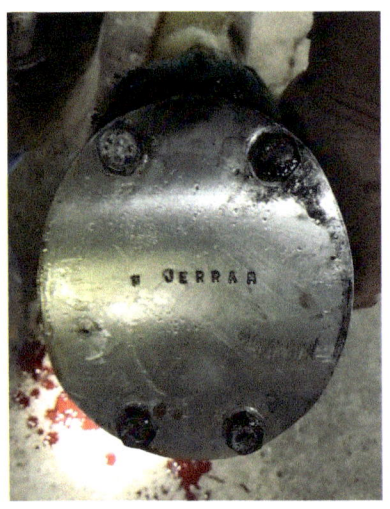

Fig. 11.12 The plate applied with 4 removable bolts.

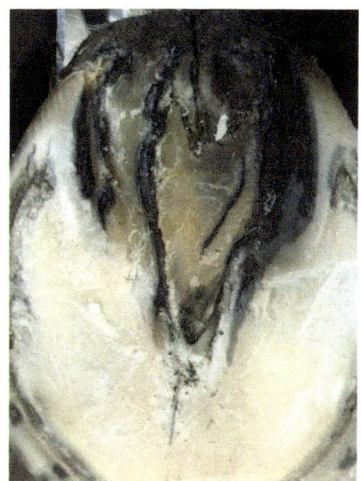

Fig. 11.14 Further progress now shows a functioning frog free from infection.

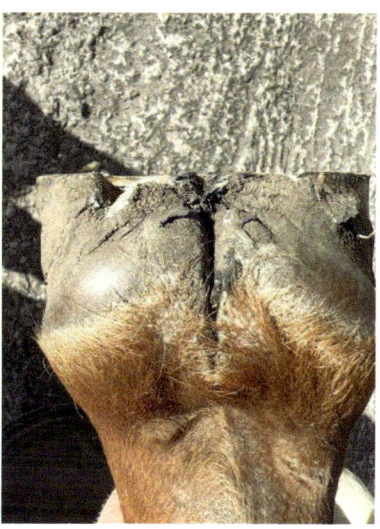

Fig. 11.15 An example of sheared heels extending the height of the frog and into the heel bulbs and skin.

Sheared heels

Sheared heels occur as a result of a split to the central sulcis of the frog that extends upwards into the heel bulbs and skin. This will lead to an independent movement of either heel with a deep cavity in the centre liable to invasion of dirt and bacteria, quite often thrush is also present (Fig. 11.15).

Consequently, there will be an imbalance of the hoof with one heel being higher than the other and an unlevel footfall. Lameness and loss of performance are often seen especially when worked in a circle.

Over time, the split can bind together with new horn developing in the previous central cavity. The heels can then no longer have independent movement and the quite often, the horse can return to soundness.

Treatment

Treatment of sheared heels often require a rebalance of the hoof with the target of level footfall being optimum. If this is not possible, then leaving the heel that is jammed up high floated is another option to allow this to relax. This is done by trimming the hoof in such a way that it doesn't make contact with the ground (Chanda et al. 2017).

Another method which is successful in the low heeled hoof is to create a spiral lift to the low side using a pad or hoof

Conditions of the frog

adhesive which can then allow the horse to land level. It is advisable with both cases to apply a bar shoe to help stop the independent movement of the heels and allow the central sulcis to regenerate. The style of bar shoe can vary and is relevant to the horse's conformation, hoof strength and environment (Fig. 11.16).

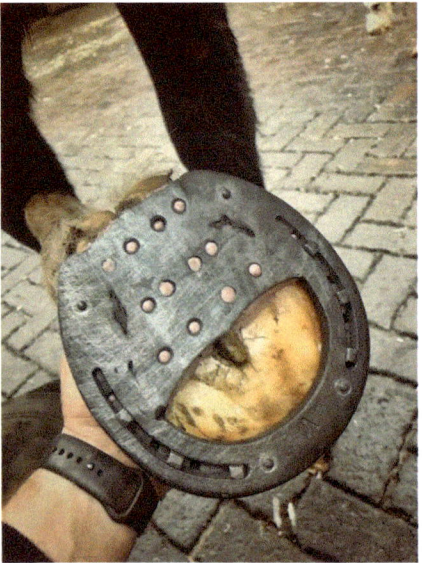

Fig. 11.16 A wide plate bar shoe that prevents the heels moving independently.

Packing of the split at the central sulcis is advisable with an anti fungal clay that can prevent any dirt entering the area, destroy any existing bacterium in the cavity and allow for regeneration of tissue in the middle of the frog (Fig.11.17).

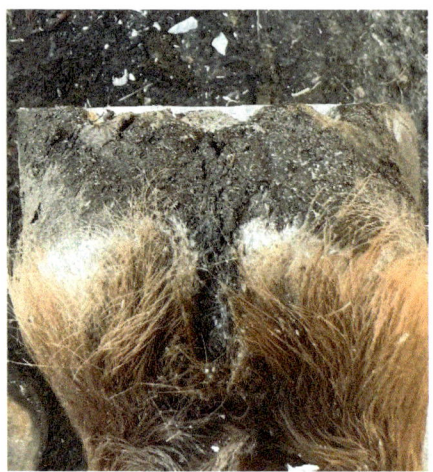

Fig. 11.17 New horn mass developed at the central sulcis resulting in the shear healing up.

Success can vary between horses, those with a more upright hoof take longer to recover due to the deep commissures of the frog having more vertical displacement during weight bearing.

Granuloma of the frog

A granuloma is a rare injury to the frog where there has been a previous wound and a large bulge had developed as it has healed (Fig. 11.18). This can be sensitive to touch and is easily bled so it is advisable that the horse's veterinarian attends to remove the granuloma and dressed accordingly to allow the area to recover. Keeping the stable clean and dry along with avoiding the use of overreach boots during recovery will speed up the healing process.

Conditions of the frog

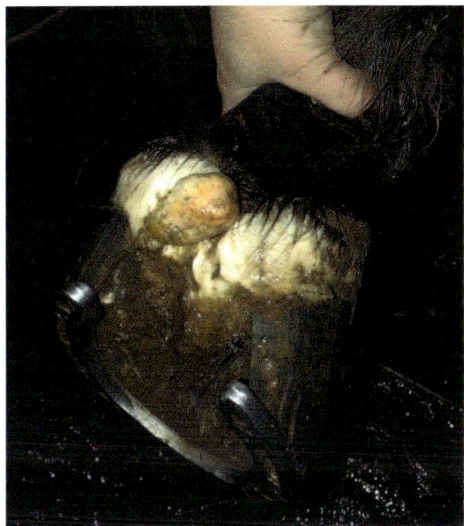

Fig. 11.18 A granuloma that has developed at the rear of the frog.

Maggot infestation of the frog

A maggot infestation can happen when there are poor hygiene conditions and lack of hoof care management. There is often a vaulted frog where flys have entered the central sulcis to lay eggs resulting in maggots (Shin et al. 2020).

There will be little to no frog to trim as a result of infestation, but if there are any pieces that are trapping maggots in then it is advisable for the farrier to remove this (Fig. 11.19). The use of diluted hydrogen peroxide applied 50:50 with water can kill maggots instantly. Repeat this for 3 days before applying less harsh treatment as the hydrogen peroxide will also destroy healthy material in time. If there is no availability of hydrogen peroxide, then the use of truck easy start spray will also destroy the infestation quickly.

Following treatment, it is advisable to assess a future plan of how to keep the stable and hooves clean to help prevent a recurrence.

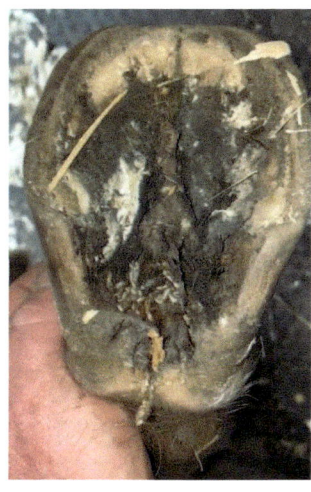

Fig. 11.19 Maggot infestation at the central sulcus of the frog.

Frog Stave

A frog stave is a piece of sharp horn that develops at the central sulcis of the frog where there has previously been a split (Fig. 11.20). The split recovers by regenerating new horn often as the result of using frog treatments, frog support pads or bar shoes. Whilst the recovery of the split is welcomed as the heels are no longer sheared, the spike of horn can create pressure on the sensitive structures at the rear of the hoof. There are also cases where heels contract as a

Conditions of the frog

result of a stave and the soft tissues above the frog get less stimulation and development.

It is recommended that this excess horn is trimmed carefully so that the body of the frog eventually becomes one smooth piece and functions as a whole.

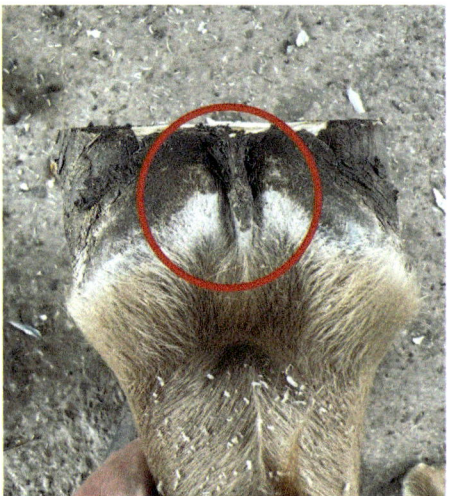

Fig. 11.20 An example of a frog stave that has developed at the central sulcus of the frog.

Exfoliating frog

Exfoliation of the frog is a natural process that takes place as new frog get developed. The entire portion of frog can come free during hoof trimming with a freshly developed frog in its place underneath. This is often a result of a prolonged dry spell of weather, where the layers of horn have compounded together to protect against hard ground. Then, after a few rain showers and the ground becoming softer, the excess horn becomes loose and peels away as one (Fig. 11.21).

This can also be the result of an infection that has under run the entirety of the frog with the corium of the frog rapidly developing new horn in response to bacterial infection and pain. If there is any bacteria present with the newly developed frog, then regular treatment with an anti fungal solution will help to encourage healthy growth.

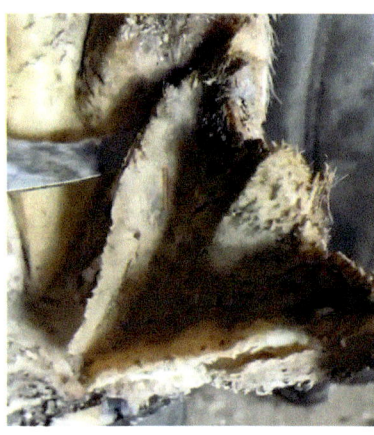

Fig. 11.21 A complete piece of frog removed as mass exfoliation following a prolonged dry spell of weather.

Atrophy of the frog

An atrophy of the frog is when the material erodes away and becomes sensitive (Fig. 11.22). This can happen to any hoof as a result of changing environmental or management conditions but is most associated with horses that are kept in dirty stables or

Conditions of the frog

deep muddy fields. Hooves that have high heels and deep clefts are also more prone to frog atrophy. Care must be taken when picking out the hoof due to the increased risk of making the frog bleed. The tip of the frog in particular will be the most compromised.

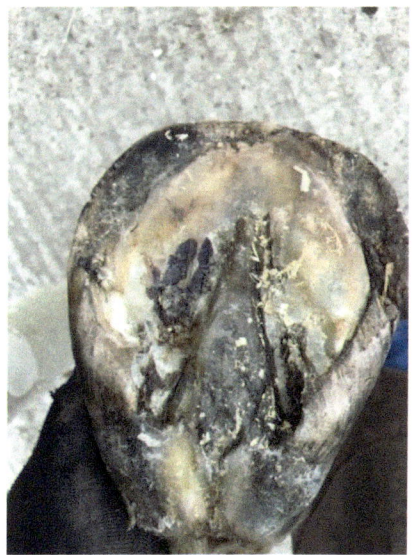

Fig. 11.22 An atrophied frog with little material to protect the sensitive structures of the hoof.

Ensuring a dry, clean stable will allow the frog to harden up but if lameness is present, pads may be required with anti fungal treatment placed under to help regenerate the layers of horn.

The effects of excessive moisture on the frog

The wetter winter months of the year bring about a change to the structure to the external hoof, most notably at the frog. This is due to being in constant contact with the wet ground during turnout and consequently the horny material of the frog can begin to soften and degrade (Fig. 11.23). Infections are more likely as bacteria can find it easier to penetrate through the material.

Whilst it is quite difficult to overcome excessive wet turnout conditions, the use of absorbent stable bedding when brought in can help to draw out any excessive moisture.

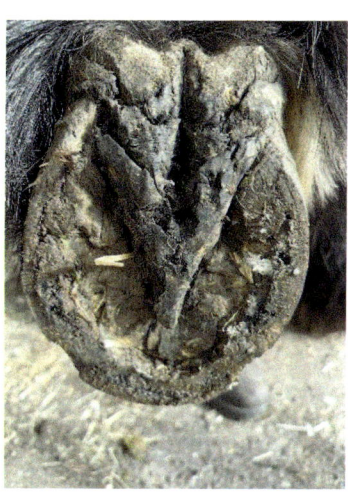

Fig. 11.23 Excessive moisture from winter turnout leading to a breakdown in the solid frog shape with a ragged appearance now present.

References

Agne, B. (2010) 'Diagnosis and treatment of foot infections' *Journal of Equine Veterinary Science*, Vol. *30*, No.9, pp 510-512.

Apprich, V., Licka, T., Zipfl, N., Tichy, A., & Gabriel, C. (2017) 'Equine hoof canker: cell proliferation and morphology' *Veterinary pathology*, Vol.*54*, No.4, pp 661-668.

Butler, D & Butler, J. (2004) '*The Principles of Horseshoeing (P3)*', Doug Butler Enterprises: Colorado, USA.

Chanda, M., Puangthong, C., Sanigavatee, K., Kiawwan, R., & Krungthongpatthana, W. (2020) 'The effect of the z-bar shoeing method on surface dimension of the hoof wall and time required for therapeutic shoeing in three horses with a sheared heel' *Journal of Applied Animal Research*, Vol. *48*, No.1, pp 406-412.

Oosterlinck, M., Deneut, K., Dumoulin, M., Gasthuys, F., & Pille, F. (2011) 'Retrospective study on 30 horses with chronic proliferative pododermatitis (canker)' *Equine Veterinary Education*, Vol. *23*, No.9, pp 466-471.

Petrov, K. K., & Dicks, L. M. (2013) 'Fusobacterium necrophorum, and not Dichelobacter nodosus, is associated with equine hoof thrush' *Veterinary microbiology*, Vol. *161*, No.3, pp 350-352.

Shin, S. K., Kim, S. M., Lioyd, S., & Cho, G. J. (2020) 'Prevalence of hoof disorders in horses in South Korea' *The Open Agriculture Journal*, Vol.*14*, No.1, pp 45-49.

* Images adapted with kind permission from Effigos AG. Hoof Explorer

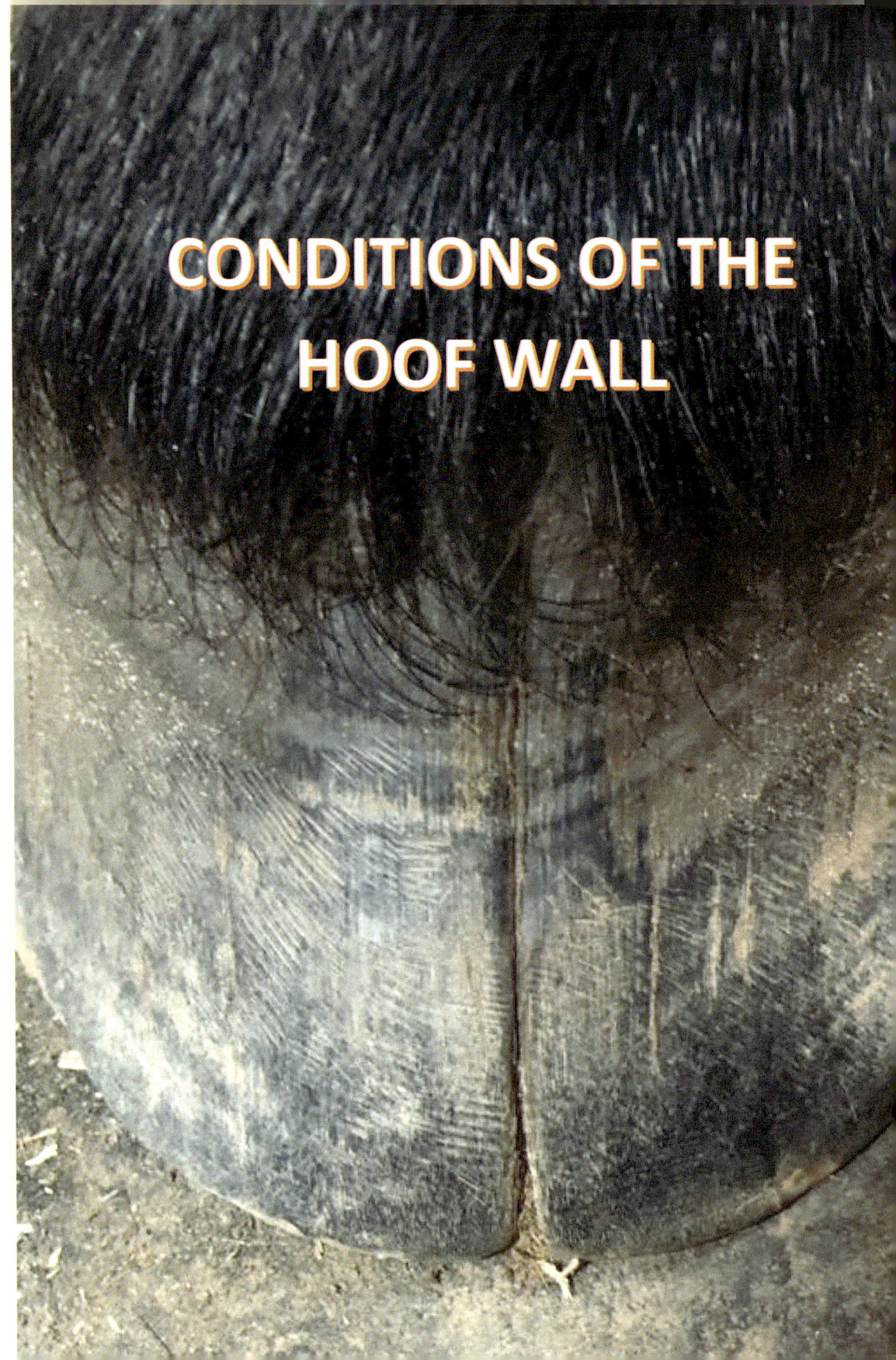

CONDITIONS OF THE HOOF WALL

Chapter 12 - Conditions of the hoof wall

Introduction

The hoof wall is the part of the hoof that is seen on the ground, it varies in height and thickness from toe to heel (Fig. 12.1). The hoof wall is made up of approximately 25% moisture with its primary function of offering protection and expansion during weight bearing.

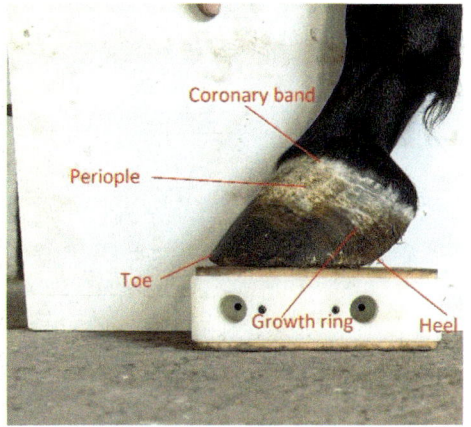

Fig 12.1 The landmark references of the hoof wall.

The hoof wall is grown at the germinative layer of the coronary corium with a hoof wall complete renewal time of 12 months as the growth descends distally. The hoof wall is attached to the pedal bone by the interdigitation of the sensitive and non sensitive laminae (Fig. 12.2).

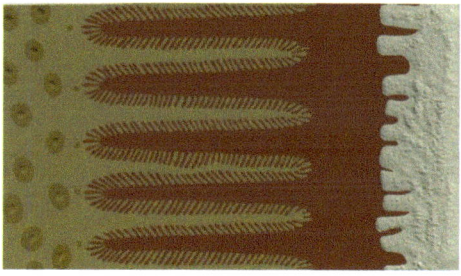

Fig. 12.2 The hoof wall attached to the pedal bone as a result of the laminal interdigitation. *

A section of hoof wall is composed of three types, these are detailed below and illustrated on the next page (Fig. 12.3):

1. Tubular horn cells – These have a multiple spiral structure which gives them strength for their function of weight bearing and shock absorption. The tubular horn cells are arranged randomly to help avoid cracks.
2. Inter tubular horn cells – This acts as a "cement" holding the tubular horn cells together in a solid mass.

Conditions of the hoof wall

3. Intra tubular horn cells – These are found within tubular horn cells and are responsible for acting as moisture conveyors enabling the horn to maintain its flexibility.

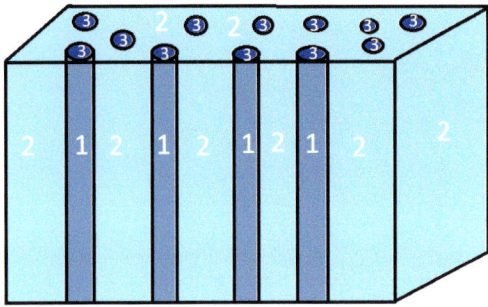

Fig. 12.3 A square section of the hoof wall with tubule arrangements.

Hoof wall cracks

Hoof wall cracks are the result of a stress or trauma to a certain area of the hoof wall (Fig. 12.4). The main categories are:

- Grass cracks
- Sand cracks
- Horizontal cracks

They are defined by their location (toe, quarter or heel), their entire length (complete or incomplete) and whether sensitive structures have been penetrated resulting in bleeding and/or infection (complicated and non complicated).

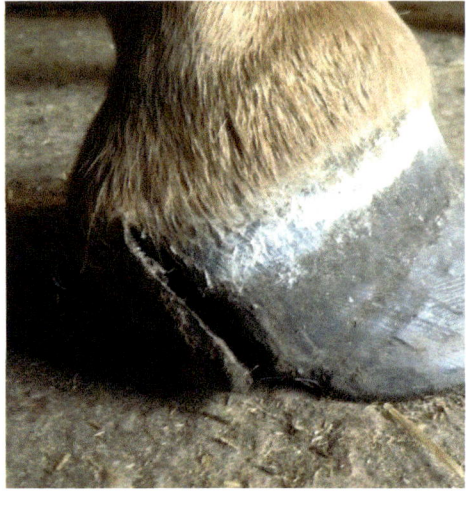

12.4 A large crack that developed on this hoof after being caught in a wire fence.

Grass cracks

Grass cracks originate from the ground and travel upwards on the hoof wall (Fig. 12.5). The crack will be opened wider at the ground surface before narrowing up and closing further up the hoof wall. This often the result of a long overgrown hoof or bacterial infection. The white line of the sole will be damaged with grit and bacteria working its way behind the crack.

Conditions of the hoof wall

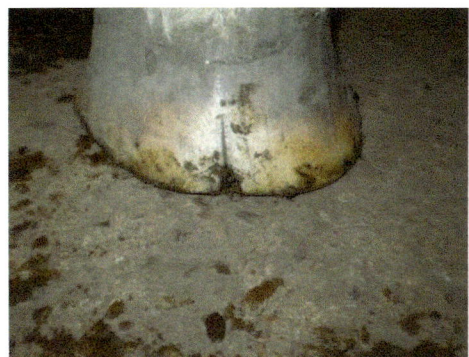

Fig. 12.5 A grasscrack originating at the base of the hoof wall.

Sand cracks

Sand cracks are often found at the quarter of the hoof but can also develop at the toe. They originate at the coronary band travel in a diagonal line down the hoof wall. This is usually the result of a hoof imbalance, conformational defaults resulting in abnormal hoof loading and the fracture point coming at the coronary band (Pardoe & Wilson, 1999). These cracks are more likely to bleed due to originating at a highly vascular area.

Toe crack

Toe cracks tend to be found in the centre of the hoof, they open up during weight bearing and the edges of the crack pinch together causing pain to the internal structures such as the sensitive laminae (Booth, 2009). If left untreated, permanent damage to the coronary corium can take place and result in a permanent deformation of new horn growth (Fig. 12.6).

The crack will need to be stabilised so that the edges can't open and close leading to pinching of the underlying sensitive structures. There are numerous methods that can be applied to achieve this, but the author has found the most success with combining a supportive bar shoe, soft setting impression material applied to the sole combined with a hoof cast (Fig. 12.7. and 12.8).

This results in new growth binding together at the coronary band and over time leads to full recovery and regeneration of a healthy hoof wall (Fig. 12.9 and 12.10).

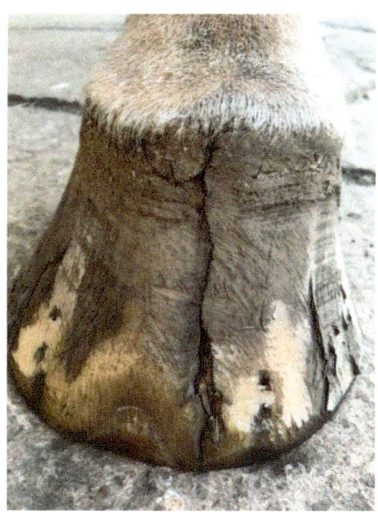

Fig. 12.6 A complete and complicated toe sandcrack resulting in lameness from the opening and closing of the crack pinching the internal sensitive structures.

Conditions of the hoof wall

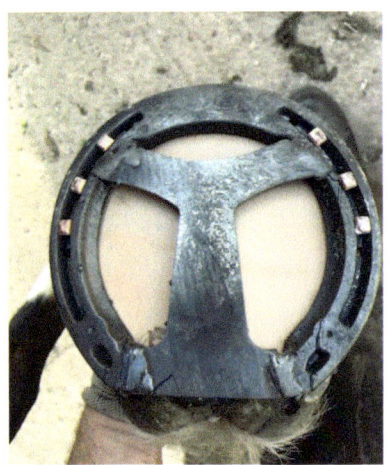

Fig. 12.7 A spider shoe combined with a leather pad created stability to the solar surface of the hoof with the leather pad dampening forces from ground contact.

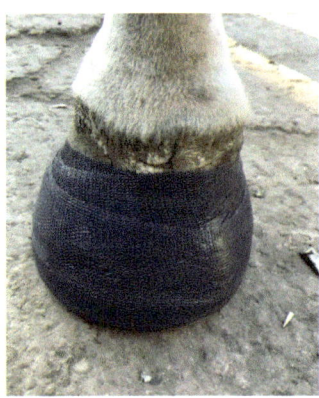

Fig. 12.8 A cast was also applied to the hoof to prevent the crack opening and closing. The top inch of hoof was left exposed to allow treatment with iodine.

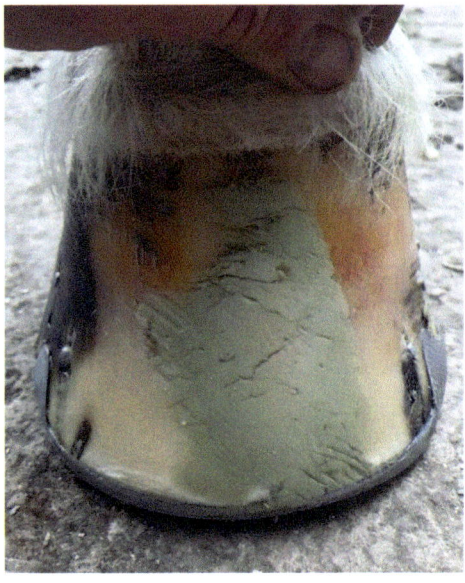

Fig. 12.9 As recovery progresses, the cast was replaced with a glue patch.

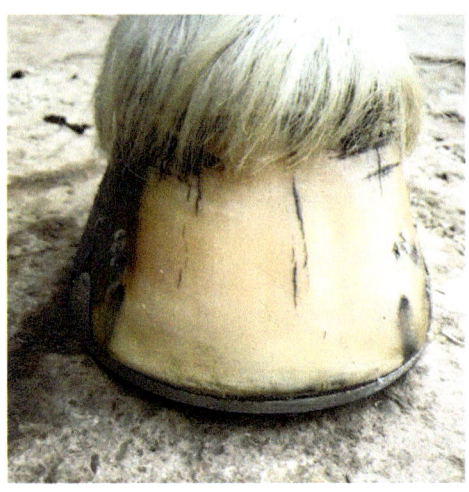

Fig. 12.10 The hoof fully rehabilitated with only minor surface cracks now present.

Conditions of the hoof wall

Quarter cracks

Quarter cracks are often the result of a medio lateral imbalance creating an uneven shift of loading forces and as a consequence the coronary band can become damaged and split (McGlinchey et al. 2020). This split can then extend downwards towards the weight bearing surface of the hoof (Fig. 12.11).

Like all cracks, the area of most movement will require immobility to heal. As the hoof expands and contracts at the quarters this can be quite challenging. The use of multiple staples that are hot branded the depth of the hoof wall can provide the most stability (Fig.12.12). This can be reinforced with hoof adhesive with a small access area to treat with anti bacterial solution if required (Fig. 12.13).

Over time, this area will begin to regenerate healthy and strong horn so that routine hoof trimming or shoeing can take its place (Fig. 12.14).

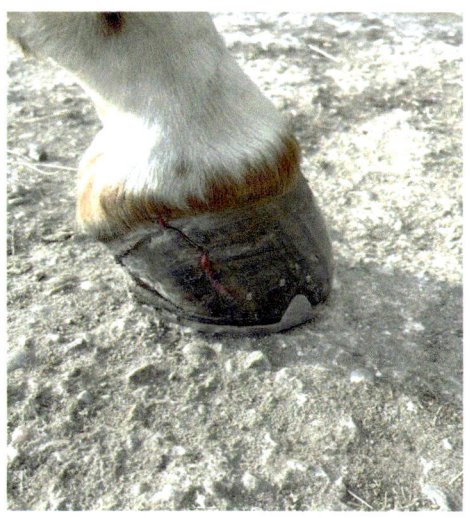

Fig. 12.11 A complicated, incomplete quarter crack that has resulted in bleeding from the coronary band. Saltwater bathing along with treatment of iodine was used for a week before there were no further signs of bleeding.

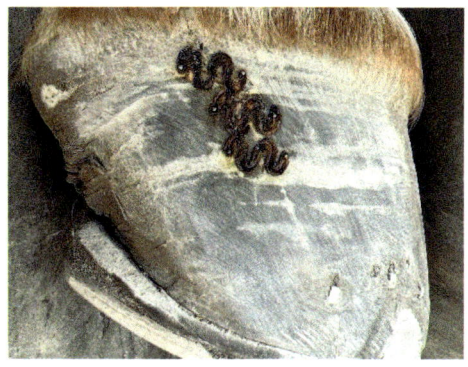

Fig. 12.12 Wire staples branded into the crack with a heat gun to stop the cracks opening and closing on weight bearing.

Conditions of the hoof wall

Horizontal cracks

Horizontal cracks occur anywhere on the hoof and are usually the result of a direct trauma or a blown out infection creating damage at the coronary band with a slit around an inch wide taking place (Fig. 12.15). As the hoof wall grows, the horizontal crack grows downwards with the hoof wall and most of the time they are stable, and therefore don't create further lameness.

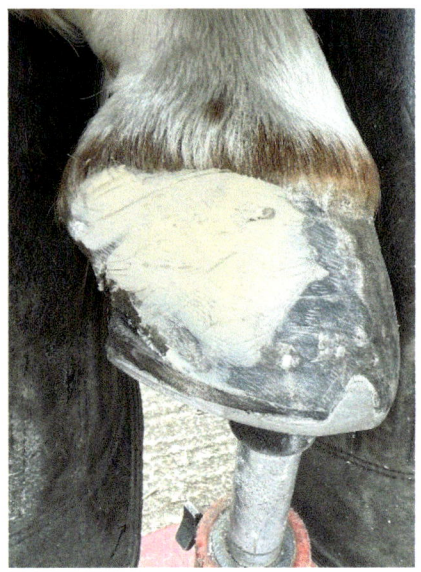

Fig. 12.13 A glue patch was applied over the staples now the crack has been treated successfully with iodine and access is no longer required.

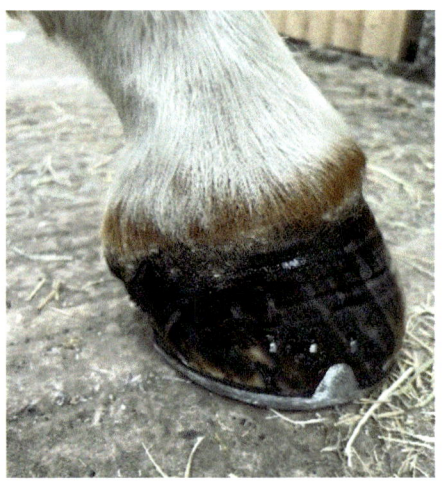

Fig. 12.14 The same hoof after a few months with no evidence of the crack.

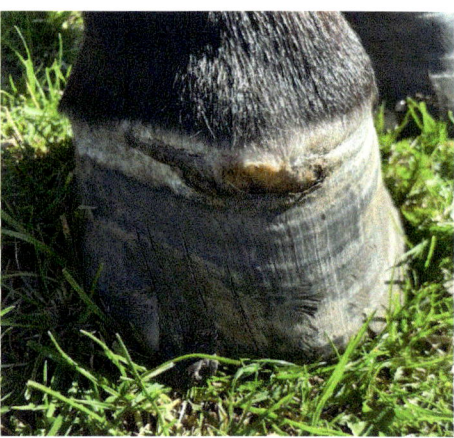

Fig. 12.15 A horizontal crack that appeared after an infection in the hoof.

Hoof avulsions

Hoof avulsions are the result of a traumatic incident resulting in a significant portion of hoof and damage to the underlying sensitive structures. There is often non weight bearing lameness and

Conditions of the hoof wall

a large amount of blood loss (Fig. 12.16 and 12.17). Taking immediate first aid action is critical to a successful outcome.

The horse's veterinarian should attend to assess the damage to the sensitive laminae and if there is any arterial damage. A clean waterproof dressing should be applied, and the horse kept on boxrest with regular cleaning out of the stable to prevent infection (Fig. 12.18).

Once this recovery time is up, the hoof can be stabilised with the use of a spider shoe to help transfer weightbearing from the area of sensitivity (Fig. 12.19). The hoof will then develop fresh new horn and eventually function normally (Fig. 12.20). There are some cases where a scarring to the coronary band can result in permanent hoof wall damage.

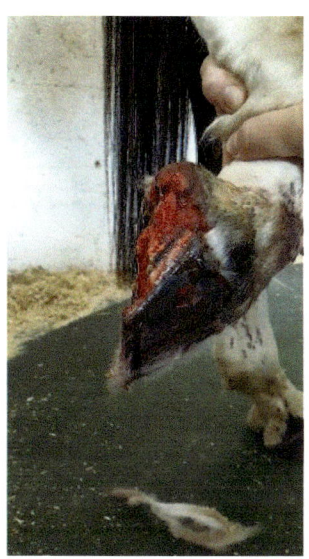

Fig. 12.17 Lateral view of the avulsion showing the full depth and amount of damage.

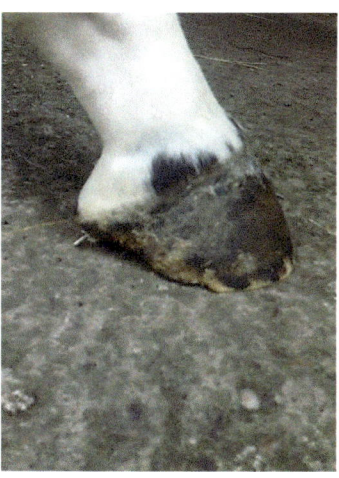

Fig. 12.18 Following box rest for a month wearing a waterproof dressing, the hoof had stabilised and is now able to be shod.

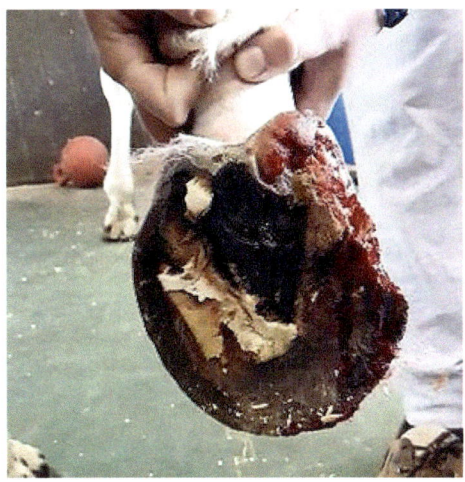

Fig. 12.16 A chronic avulsion to a hind foot.

Conditions of the hoof wall

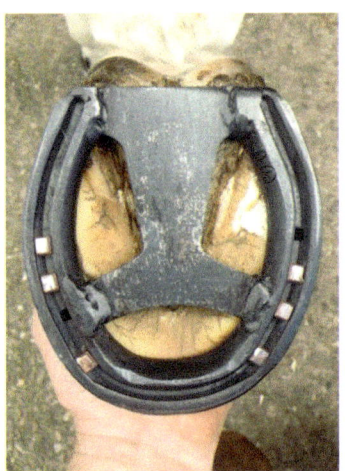

Fig. 12.19 A spider shoe was applied to take weight and loading forces away from the damaged area and transfer to the frog and opposite branch.

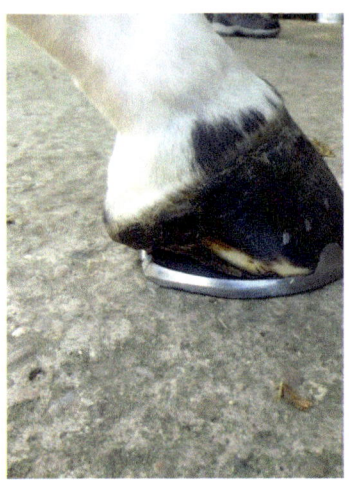

Fig. 12.20 The hoof now looking far less damaged, the horse returned to full soundness.

Tread

A tread is the name given to an injury of the coronary band caused by a shoe on the opposite hoof. This can happen when turning, working at speed or as a result of an accident whilst travelling on a horse box (Fig. 12.21). Treads occur most frequently when horses are shod with sharp edges or when wearing screw in jumping studs.

The level of damage can range from bruising to an open wound. If an open wound is present, veterinary advice should be sought due to the risk of an infection developing and possibly a false quarter. An assessment of the horse's medio lateral balance should be considered along with fitting shoes with all sharp edges removed. The use of protective boots may be required when the horse is in work or travelling.

Conditions of the hoof wall

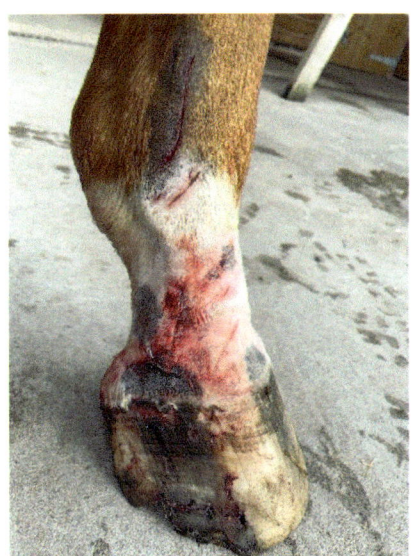

Fig. 12.21 Injury to the coronary band and lower limb as a result of a tread injury after a traumatic journey in a trailer.

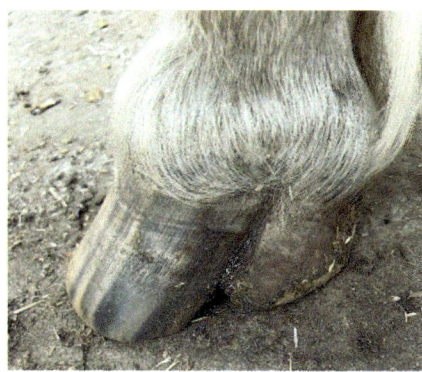

Fig. 12.22 A false quarter that has developed from an old wire injury to the coronary band.

False quarter

A false quarter is the name given to a vertical indentation in the hoof wall parallel to the horn tubules. These are not true cracks but develop as a result of damage to the coronary band from wire injuries or penetration from sharp objects (Fig. 12.22). As long as the underlying sensitive structures are not involved, then specialised shoeing is not required. Due to the damage at the coronary band, the defect in the hoof will be permanent. Quite often, the horn around the false quarter will be weak and not provide adequate security for nailing so special consideration should be taken when placing the nailholes in the fitted shoe.

Keratoma

A keratoma is a benign tumour that develops at the inner aspect of the hoof wall and sometimes the sole. The tumour consists of hard horn either cylindrical or spherical in shape that can extend varying distances up the hoof wall. This tumour will deflect the white line inwards, as the tumour increases in size, lameness will develop (Fig. 12.23). A radiograph will reveal a defect in the coffin bone caused by pressure from the keratoma (Fig. 12.24). A keratoma can also make the hoof prone to recurrent solar abscesses even in the cleanest of environments.

Conditions of the hoof wall

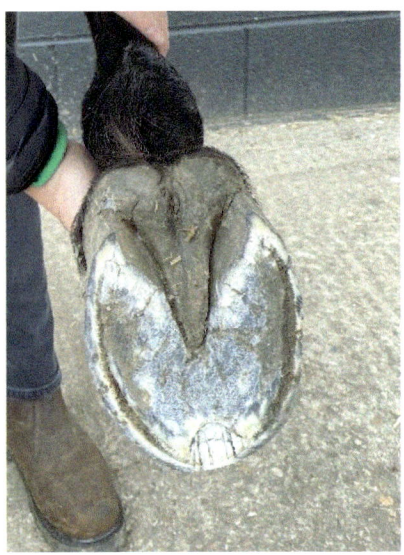

Fig. 12.23 The white line deflected inwards at the toe as a result of a keratoma.

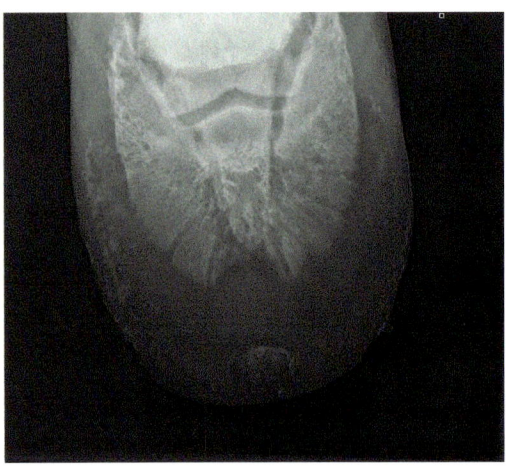

Fig. 12.24 A radiograph showing a notch of the pedal bone missing as a result of a keratoma eroding the bone.

Causes

- Repetitive concussion
- Coronary band injury
- Sandcracks
- Direct trauma

Treatment

The tumour will most likely need to be removed for a successful outcome. This will be performed at an equine hospital under general anaesthetic (Fig. 12.25). A portion of the hoof wall is removed with a cutting disc before the tumour cells are debrided with a scalpel. Post surgery, the horse will require a hospital plate shoe and protective wrap to keep the avulsion clean and prevent infection. Once the cavity has grown out, standard trimming or shoeing can be applied.

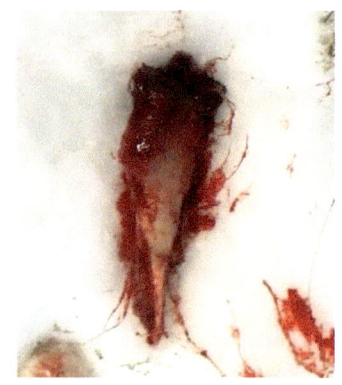

Fig. 12.25 A keratoma removed by surgery using a cutting disc to enter through the hoof wall and scalpel to remove the tumour tissue.

Prognosis

If all aspects of the tumour are removed, then complete recovery is possible. It may be necessary in some cases to provide additional protection to the hoof with bar shoes or pads if the sole and/or hoof wall have become unstable. Failure to successfully stabilise the avulsion can result in lameness similar to a complicated hoof wall crack (Fig. 12.26).

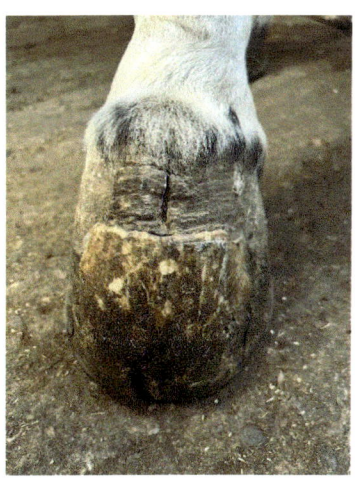

Fig. 12.26 A complicated toe sand crack developing as a result of the glue on aluminium plate failing to fully stabilise the hoof following keratoma surgery.

Coronitis

Coronitis is a rare inflammation of the coronary band that effects the quality of the periople produced and often results in bleeding wounds (Menzies-Gow et al. 2002). The chestnuts and ergots are sometimes also affected as a result with similar symptoms shown in that area (Fig. 12.27).

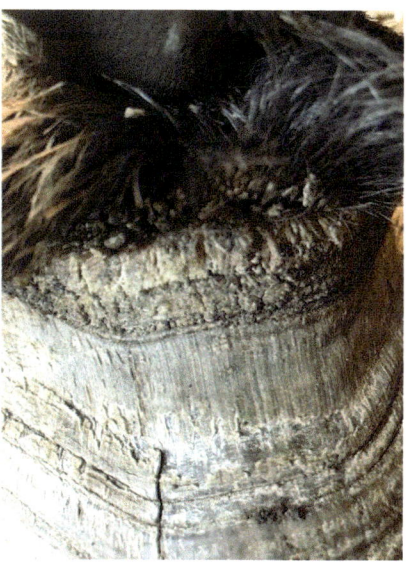

Fig. 12.27 Inflammation to the coronary band that has also resulted in an excess of chalky horn and bleeding tissue.

Growth rings

Growth rings refer to ripples on the exterior surface of the hoof wall. They can vary in size, shape and location. There are many times that growth rings are confused with a laminitic episode, but they can occur for a variety of reasons such as a change of diet from a low sugar to high sugar pasture or from excessive concussion. Laminitic growth rings tend

Conditions of the hoof wall

to diverge towards the heel as a result of the coffin bone rotating (Fig. 12.28).

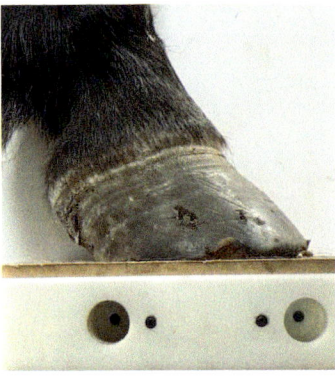

Fig. 12.28 Diverging growth rings in a laminitic pony, note the curvature towards the heel as a result of directional pull of the deep digital flexor tendon.

They don't cause lameness but indicate a change in the horse's hoof growth due to the hoof wall being developed at the coronary corium which is located within the coronary band (Fig. 12.29 and 12.30).

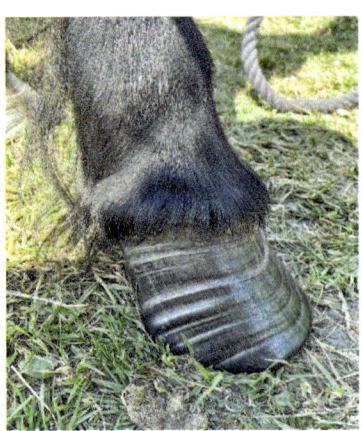

Fig. 12.29 Growth rings on the hoof wall of a feral exmoor pony.

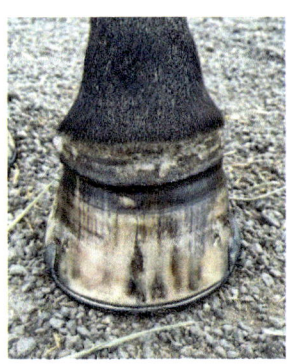

Fig. 12.30 A prominent growth ring on a rescued horse that was malnourished and began a period of weight gain.

Hoof wall bruising

The hoof wall can occasionally present with a red stain that resembles a bruise, particularly if the hoof wall is white (Fig. 12.31). This is often a result of direct trauma, excessive moisture, post operation trauma, a pressure point from hoof growth or recovery from infection or laminitis (Fig. 12.32). Hoof wall bruises don't tend to cause lameness in the same way a sole bruise would and therefore no treatment is required other than to maintain a regular trimming cycle and a healthy diet.

Conditions of the hoof wall

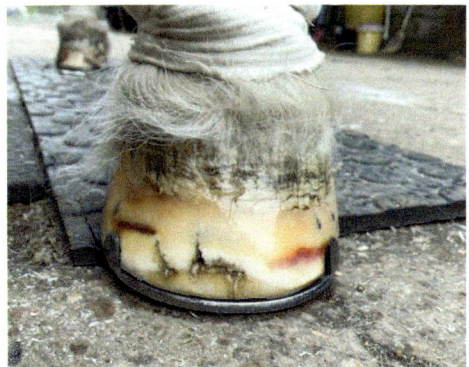

Fig. 12.31 Hoof wall bruising in a recovering laminitis case. Note the bruising is not sensitive for the horse.

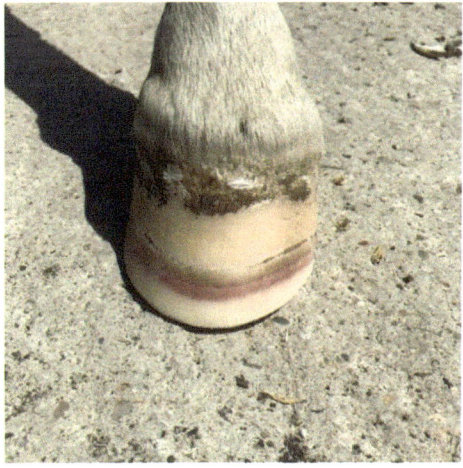

Fig. 12.32 A band of bruising that originally developed at the coronary band following a leg fracture.

Vermin damage

Damage to the hoof wall and coronary band can occur when there is a rat infestation at the stable yard. There are often gouges taken out of the hoof wall and in some instances bleeding at the softer coronary band (Fig. 12.33). It is advisable to humanely destroy the vermin infestation in order to restore hoof health as any topical dressings may not have the desired effect to prevent rats wanting to digest the horn.

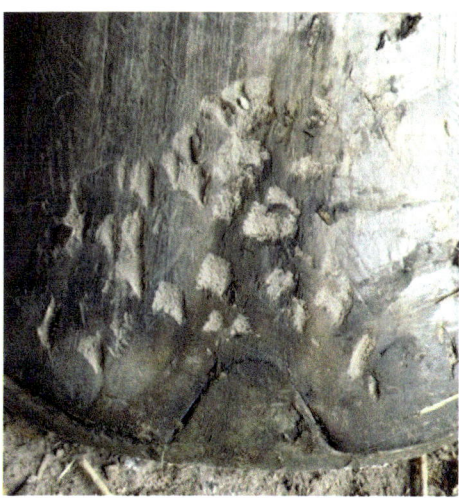

Fig. 12.33 A hoof wall showing signs of damage from rats biting the horn.

Solar Crena Marginilis

Solar crena marginilis more commonly referred to as a crena. This is a small defect in the hoof wall and white line, usually at the toe and is often confused with a grass crack (Fig. 12.34). This small crack is a result of a breakdown of a small section of the laminal interdigitation from the invasion of bacteria and foreign bodies (Fig. 12.35).

Conditions of the hoof wall

A crena can occur in both shod and unshod horses with a small notch out of the pedal bone in long term cases. The most successful method of treatment is to apply antiseptic spray to the area and maintain a regular trimming schedule to ensure the hoof wall doesn't distort further and allow more bacteria to penetrate the area.

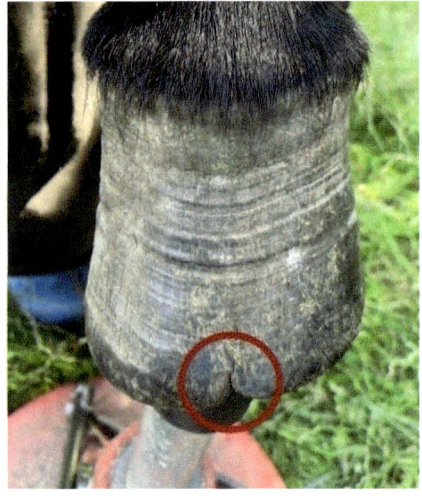

Fig. 12.34 A crena at the toe of the hoof wall (circled).

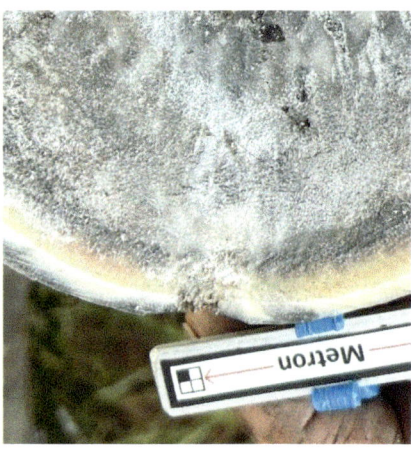

Fig. 12.35 Inward deflection of the hoof wall and degradation of the white line.

Hoof wall separation syndrome (HWSS)

Hoof wall separation syndrome (HWSS) is a genetic condition that results in peeling and shedding of the hoof wall layers even when environmental and management conditions are optimal (Fig. 12.36).

HWSS is often associated with the Connemara but can be seen in other breeds. Over a long period of time, lameness can develop due to the malfunction of the hoof (Moyer, 2003). At present there are no known cures or medication to help with this condition other than good management. Short term solutions such as hoof casts or boots can provide comfort and relief to the hoof but doesn't resolve the underlying condition (Fig. 12.37).

Conditions of the hoof wall

The Connemara breeds have a test that can be taken to see if the pony is likely to pass on the condition to their offspring as carriers or if they are indeed positive for the gene.

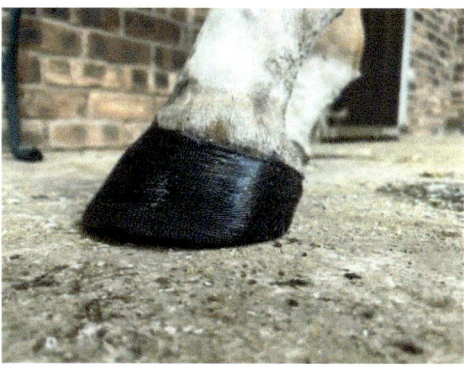

Fig. 12.37 A hoof cast applied to provide relief to the sensitive hoof and allow the horse to walk around comfortably.

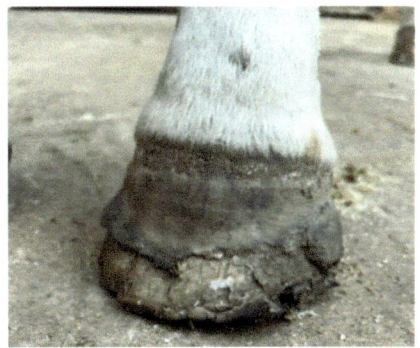

Fig. 12.36 A case of HWSS resulting in a peeling of the hoof wall. Attempts at gluing on a shoe proved to be unsuccessful.

Concussive trauma to the hoof wall

Concussive trauma to the hoof wall can result in a splitting and separation of the lower aspect of the hoof wall and most notably at the heel region (Fig. 12.38). The upper hoof wall remains unaffected and secure nailing of shoes is still possible. This is often caused by a hard arena surface or road work on hooves that are genetically weak or heels that are low due to long sloping pasterns.

Working the horse on a softer arena surface with reduce the damage caused but if this is not possible then the use of leather pads combined with packing made up of leather shreds coated in anti bacterial solution can provide a dampening effect against the surfaces worked on (Fig. 12.39). Over time, the damaged area will recover, and hoof quality can improve.

Conditions of the hoof wall

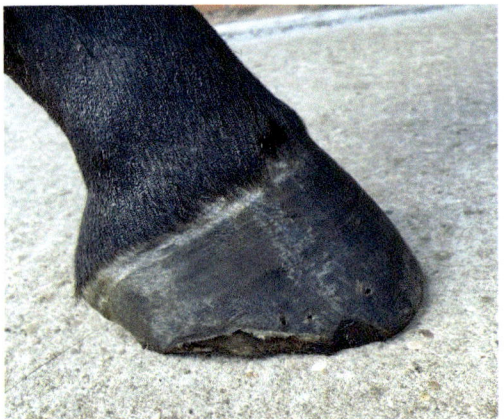

Fig. 12.38 *The lower portion of the hoof showing damage from excessive concussion.*

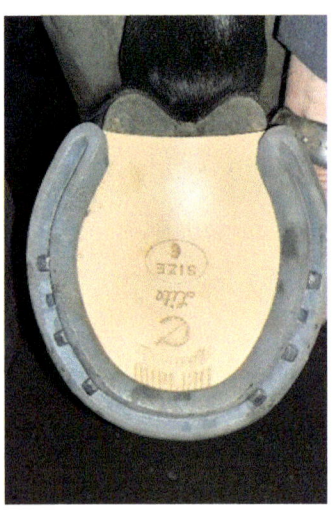

Fig. 12.39 *A leather pad applied to dampen concussive forces on the hoof.*

Excessive Periople

There can be times of excessive moisture or dry weather can result in a thickening and increase in the amount of Periople on the top of the hoof wall (Fig. 12.40). This does not impede hoof function and it is advisable not to try to remove this layer as it helps to regulate moisture absorption from the environment. As weather conditions change, the Periople will adapt in accordance to protect the coronary band and the upper third of the hoof wall.

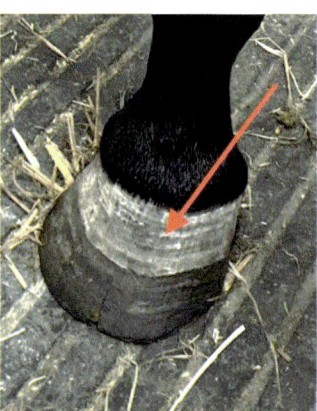

Fig. 12.40 *Prominent Periople on a dry hoof.*

References

Booth, T. (2009) 'Clinical aspects of the equine foot Part 3: Hoof cracks and wall injury' *UK Vet Companion Animal*, Vol. *14, No.*2, pp 5-10.

Butler, D & Butler, J. (2004) '*The Principles of Horseshoeing (P3)*', Doug Butler Enterprises: Colorado, USA.

McGlinchey, L., Robinson, P., Porter, B., Sidhu, A. B. S., & Rosanowski, S. M. (2020) 'Quarter cracks in Thoroughbred racehorses trained in Hong Kong over a 9-year period (2007-2015): incidence, clinical presentation, and future racing performance' *Equine Veterinary Education*, Vol. *32*, pp 18-24.

Menzies-Gow, N. J., McGowan, C. M., Patterson-Kane, J. C., & Bond, R. (2002) 'Coronary band dystrophy in two horses' *Veterinary record*, Vol. *150, No.*21, pp 665-668.

Moyer, W. (2003) 'Hoof wall defects: chronic hoof wall separations and hoof wall cracks' *Veterinary Clinics: Equine Practice*, Vol. *19, No.* 2, pp 463-477.

Pardoe, C. H., & Wilson, A. M. (1999) 'In vitro mechanical properties of different equine hoof wall crack fixation techniques' *Equine veterinary journal*, Vol. *31,* No.6, pp 506-509.

* Images adapted with kind permission from Effigos AG. Hoof Explorer

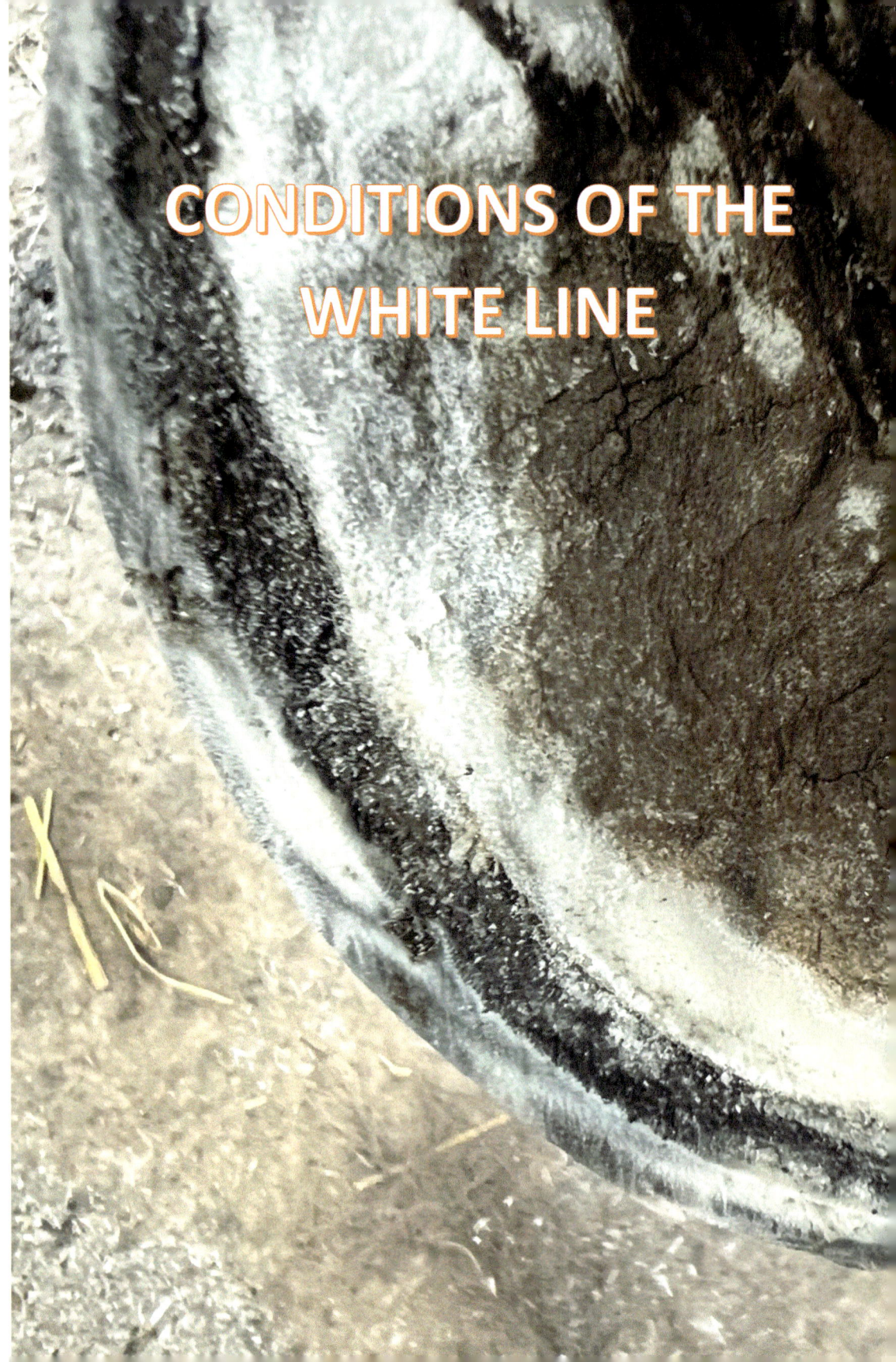

CONDITIONS OF THE WHITE LINE

Conditions of the white line

Chapter 13 - Conditions of the white line

Introduction

The white line is the junction between the sole and hoof wall (Fig 13.1). The white line is developed at the terminal papillae of the sensitive laminae and fills in the spaces between the non sensitive laminae. This then forms an irregular line around the inner aspect of the hoof wall when viewed at the sole and is usually around 3mm wide.

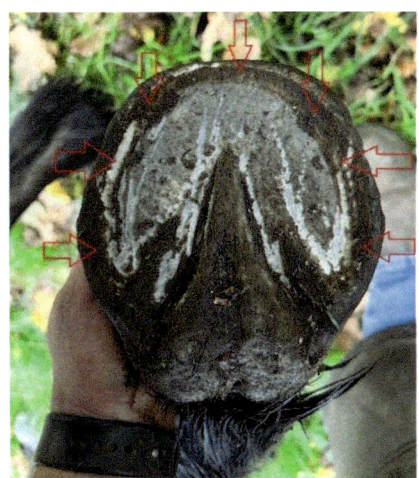

Fig 13.1 The white line (red arrows) of the hoof that acts as a junction between the sole and hoof wall.

The horn produced is not pigmented and therefore gets termed as "white line".

The white line contains around 50% moisture which aids its function of absorbing concussion when the hoof wall moves outwards during weight bearing and the sole flattens.

Abscess

An abscess is a bacterial infection of the hoof which normally occurs in the white line of the hoof due the ease of penetration in this area for bacteria from the environment. Liquefactive necrosis causes pus formation sometimes with gas accumulation within the hoof capsule. Pus is a mixture of tissue fluid, white blood cells, cellular debris & bacteria (Cole et al. 2019).

Abscesses are defined by their location, sub-solar is an infection in the solar corium whilst sub-mural is an infection behind the hoof wall. The infection will follow the path of least resistance and break out either at the white line of the sole or at the coronary due to its flexible structure (Fig. 13.2 and 13.3). Lameness can vary from mild to severe but in most cases, there is an increased digital pulse along with heat in the hoof.

Conditions of the white line

The infections are categorised into two types, depending on the structures involved:

- Grade 1 infection- This a less severe infection, only soft tissues are involved and is considered superficial although they may be a separation of the sensitive tissues.

- Grade 2 infection – This is a more serious deep infection involving other structures within the hoof such as the bursae, joint capsule & bone.

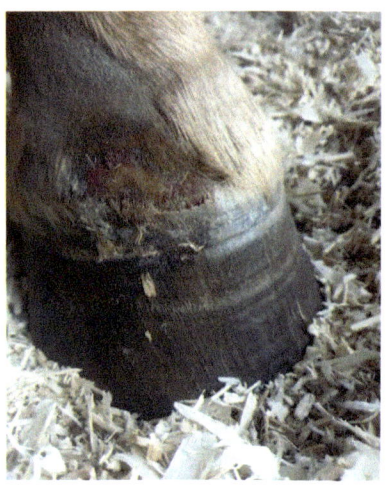

Fig. 13.3 An abscess that has drained at the coronary band.

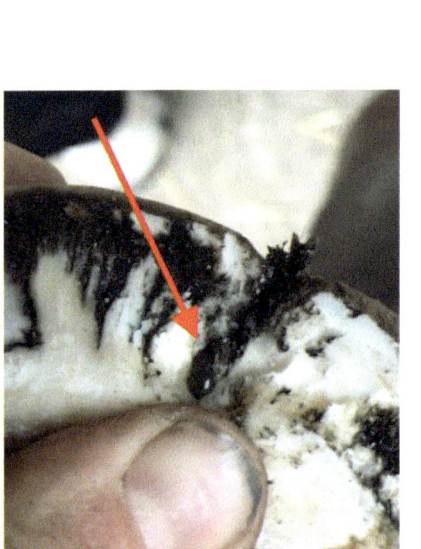

Fig. 13.2 An abscess that has begun draining at the white line in the toe. Note the black liquid discharge.

Causes

The main reasons for the infection to develop are:

- Bacterial infection/puncture wound.
- Gravel trapped in the white line.
- Nail bind.
- Nail prick.
- Dirty stable conditions.
- Poor quality grazing land.
- Changeable wet and dry conditions trapping bacteria in the hoof.

Conditions of the white line

Treatment

Abscesses can be located using hoof testers and trimming the sole. Once the pus pocket has been breached, drainage is then initiated and the horse experiences instant relief. A hot poultice is then applied to the hoof with daily saltwater bathing during a dressing change. This should be performed daily until all pus is drained and the horse's soundness begins to improve (Trayhorn, 2019).

The process of how to apply a poultice

A poultice is a wrap applied to the hoof to help draw out any bacterial material and to help relieve pressure if an infection hasn't been drained yet. It is advisable to change the dressing daily with hot saltwater bathing in a bucket in between dressing changes.

There are multiple methods and materials that can be used to achieve this so this guide will be a description of what the author has found to be successful over many years in dealing with hoof infections.

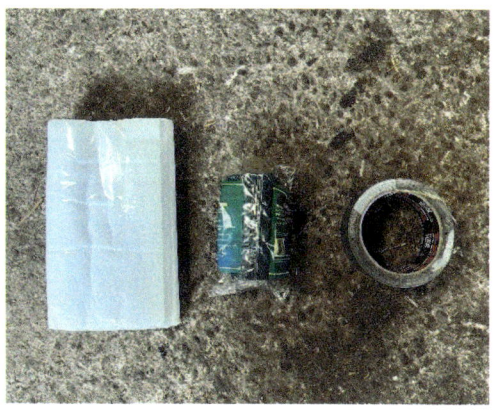

1. *The three main components in order of application from left to right: Intex packing, vet wrap and industrial tape.*

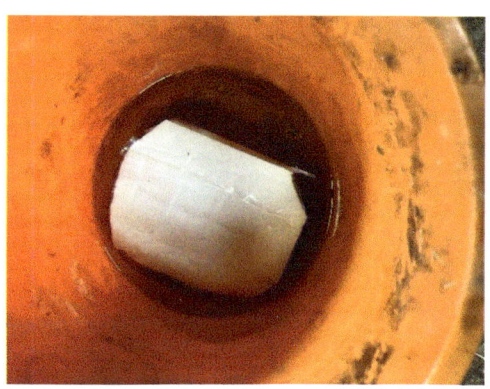

2. *Cut the intex pad to the size and shape of the solar surface of the hoof then soak in boiling hot water. Alternatively, for smaller hooves it is possible to use a child's nappy to attach to the hoof which will help draw out infection.*

Conditions of the white line

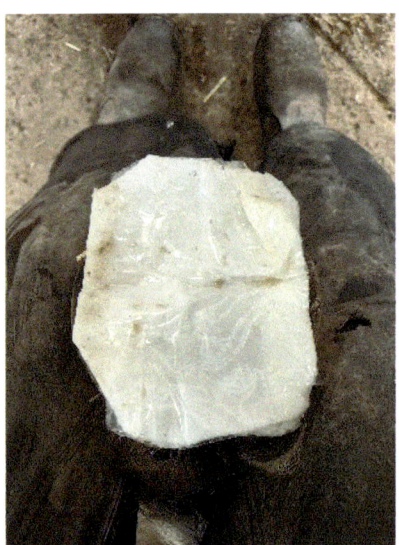

3. The soaked intex is laid on the hoof. The shiny plastic layer should be facing you.

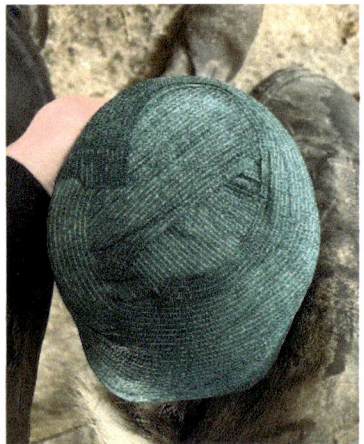

4. The vet wrap is then wrapped around the intex and the whole hoof to hold it in position. As the vet wrap can bind to itself, it possible to place the hoof on a clean dry floor if you need a break from holding the hoof up. Ensure the whole hoof is wrapped for the tightest security.

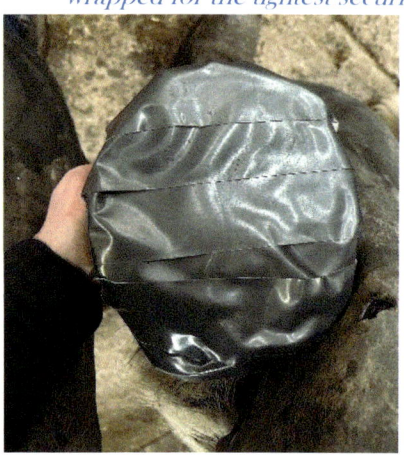

5. Industrial tape is wrapped around the dressing to provide a waterproof layer.

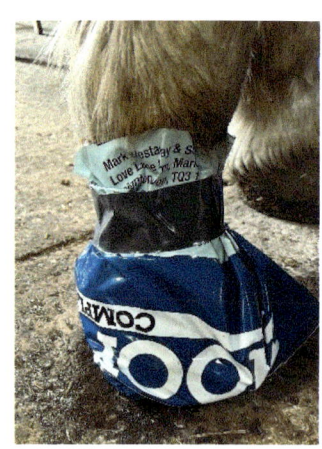

6. A plastic feedbag can also be used as a further waterproof layer with a wrap of tape around the pastern to hold it in position.

Conditions of the white line

This is particularly useful for horses that don't settle on box rest.

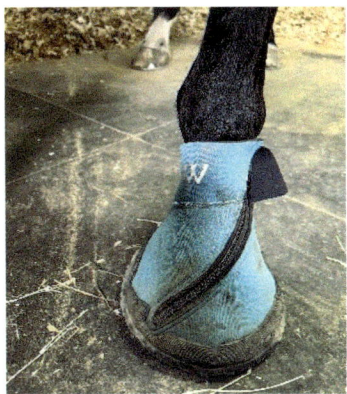

7. *Alternatively, a zip up poultice boot can be used for daily dressing and is robust enough for hand walking the horse if required.*

Once the horse has become sound, a shoe can then be applied with a protective pad and anti fungal clay to provide protection to a sensitive area whilst also eliminating any existing or potential bacteria.

If dressing to a puncture wound is still required, a hospital plate can be applied to allow access to change dressings whilst protecting the sole. Once the puncture is resolved, a normal shoe can then be applied.

Over time, there may be an under run sole develop that will result in the whole sole coming off with a fresh new sole underneath, this may be softer than the previous sole due to lack of interaction with the ground so it may be advisable to apply pads as a protective layer as the sole thickens up again (Fig. 13.4).

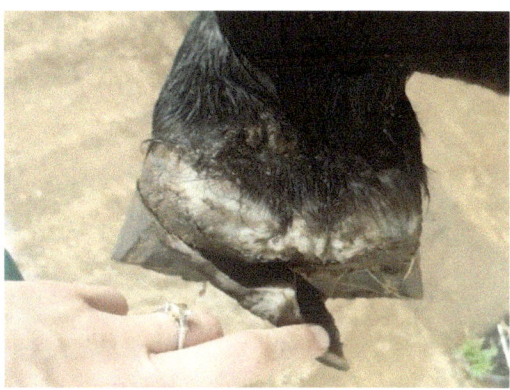

Fig. 13.4 An under run sole and frog that has come away after a large infection to the sole.

White line disease

White line disease (also known as Onycomycosis) is a fungal infection of the stratum medium (inner hoof wall). This can be described as a keratolytic process in the solear surface of the hoof (Fig. 13.5). White line disease occurs when the white line becomes stretched from either leverage forces from a flared hoof wall or from debris becoming wedged in the white line making it easier for bacteria to then enter the area. Horn digesting fungi such as *Psudoallscheria boydii* and *Scopulariopsis* thrive in dark wet environments which are typical of the horse's hoof.

Conditions of the white line

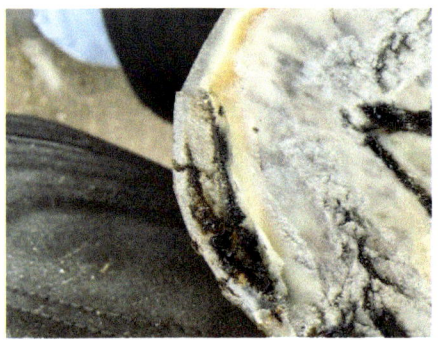

Fig. 13.5 Separation of the white line with bacteria present.

The infected area is soft and has a degraded, cheesy appearance. This usually originates at the quarter and migrates round to the toe as the infection progresses in contrast to seedy toe which is usually limited to the toe region. There are two microorganisms known as heterotrophs and saprophytes that exist in a symbiotic relationship and become embedded in the hoof wall (Kuwano et al. 1998). They then produce thread like filaments known as hyphae that absorb nutrients. The stratum medium is digested by the invading organisms which break down the cross linking keratin molecules. Lameness rarely occurs until the disease is at an advanced stage resulting in a hoof wall that will struggle to hold a shoe.

Causes

Microorganisms do not attack healthy hoof, so they usually gain entry via a hoof crack or fissure at the white line (Fig. 13.6). Other factors include:

- Acute trauma
- Abscess or infection
- Laminitis that creates tears in the stratum medium of the hoof (Dense hoof wall).
- Solar bruising near the white line. Dried blood provides growth nutrients for the causative organism.
- Bad stable conditions – Manure can extract keratin that binds hoof horn together.

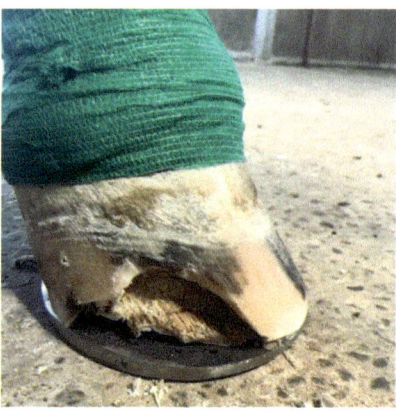

Fig 13.6 An area of white line disease infection that has been removed by hoof nippers, knife and a motorised burr.

Treatment

The infected area should be debrided using farriery tools before then using a motorised burr to help tidy up the edges of the infection so that all diseased material has been removed. The

Conditions of the white line

avulsion can now be cleaned daily using an antiseptic solution. The hoof may require extra stability in the form of a heart bar shoe to help unload the weakened side of the hoof (Fig. 13.7).

application can be used for treatment whilst helping to keep a shoe on for a full cycle (Fig. 13.8).

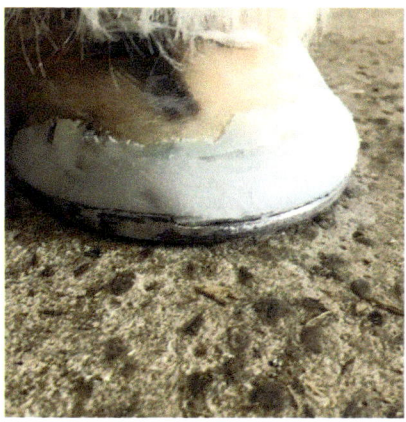

Fig. 13.8 A copper sulphate infused thermoplastic patch applied to the medial side of a hoof with white line disease.

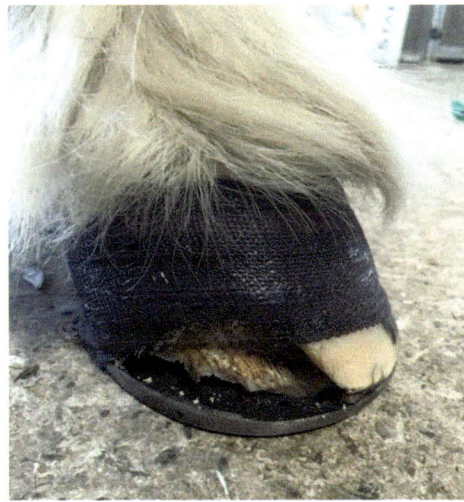

Fig. 13.7 A heart bar shoe has been applied to this hoof to help provide stability to a weakened hoof along with a hoof cast with a window cut open to allow for daily treatment.

There may be some cases of white line disease that involve the medial aspect of the hoof resulting in a large cavity that makes shoe attachment and retainment difficult because of the risk of the horse stepping off the shoe. This can be overcome by filling the cavity with a thermoplastic patch glued to the hoof wall. Placing the thermoplastic in a pot of copper sulphate powder prior to

Prognosis

There will need to be a big change in the horse's daily management with increased hoof picking, thicker and more absorbent stable bedding long with an increase of mucking out to ensure bacteria is kept to a minimum. If all the above criteria are achieved, the chances of a full recovery are high.

Seedy toe

Seedy toe is a similar hoof infection to white line disease but is confined to the toe area of the hoof. The bacteria *Candida albicans* creates a yeast infection of the inner third of the hoof wall. The toe of the hoof wall becomes weak and filled with mealy and crumbly horn.

There will be a persistent cavity at the toe as a result of separation between the sensitive and non sensitive laminae, this usually occurs as a result of a laminitic episode as the laminae in his region have become damaged from a haematoma as a result of trauma (Fig. 13.9). The separation that then develops makes it easier for bacteria to penetrate the hoof. It has been reported that 43.5% of horses aged over 30 have widened white lines and that 14.5% have developed seedy toe which may explain its prevalence in the veteran horse (Moyer, 2003).

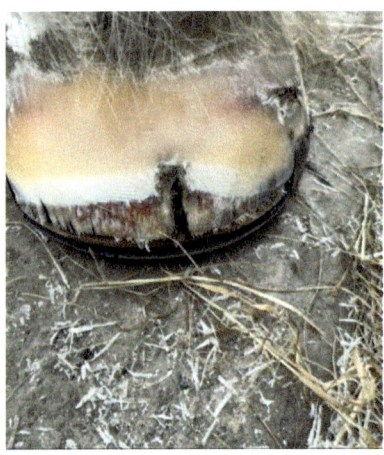

Fig. 13.9 A seedy toe infection as a result of laminitis.

Causes

Seedy toe infection can be caused by:

- Laminitis – As a result of the breakdown of the laminal interdigitation.

- Poor stable management.

- Poor quality grazing land.

- Failure to pick out feet resulting in a harvest of bacteria.

Treatment

Regular farriery appointments will prevent the hoof from becoming distorted and white line stretched as this could result in an increase of bacterial penetration. The exposed seedy toe is treated daily with an antiseptic spray whilst being housed in a clean dry moisture absorbing bedding.

Prognosis

Although lameness is rarely observed, seedy toe can be a difficult infection to completely clear up due to the breakdown of the laminal interdigitation so therefore the chances of complete recovery are guarded.

Gravel tracks

Gravel tracks are the result of stones and grit entering the white line on a barefoot hoof, this does not tend to happen in the

Conditions of the white line

shod hoof due to protection of the white line that a shoe can offer (Fig. 13.10). It most commonly occurs during prolonged dry spells when stones get wedged in the hoof from being led or ridden down hard and rough surfaces. The result is a cavity that can range from being small to being the complete length of hoof wall (DeBowes & Yovich, 1989).

There is an increased risk of an abscess or white line disease forming due to the invasion of bacteria into the cavity. Cases that involve the full length of the hoof wall may require a resection of the hoof to successfully eliminate bacteria and allow healthy horn to regenerate (Ireland et al. 2012).

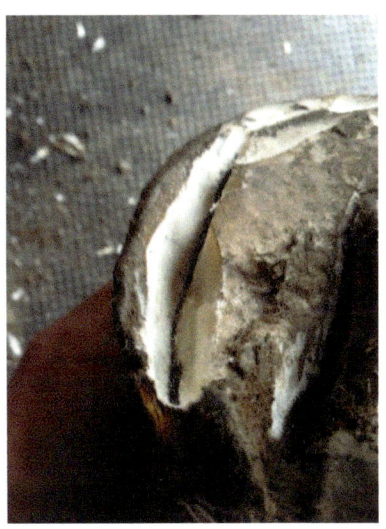

Fig. 13.10 A deep cavity in the hoof as a result of gravel becoming wedged.

Treatment

In some cases, it may be necessary to radiograph the hoof to determine the depth and size of the cavity before hoof trimming (Fig. 13.11). The cavity should be excavated and cleaned prior to packing with an antiseptic putty (Fig. 13.12).

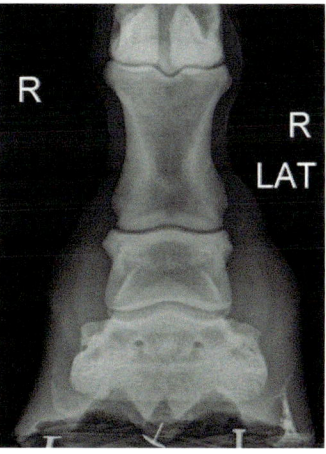

Fig. 13.11 A radiograph showing damage to the white line with a white shadow on the right side of the image which is made up of gravel material.

Conditions of the white line

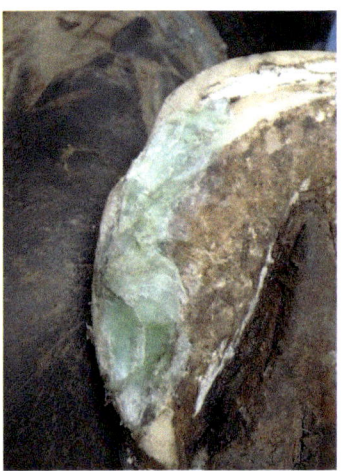

Fig. 13.12 The cavity is packed with keratex anti septic putty.

This is more successful when applied under a shoe to help hold the putty in place until the cavity has eventually grown out (Fig. 13.13). Once the cavity is gone, it is possible to return to barefoot if required or remain shod if the horse's workload and environment requires this.

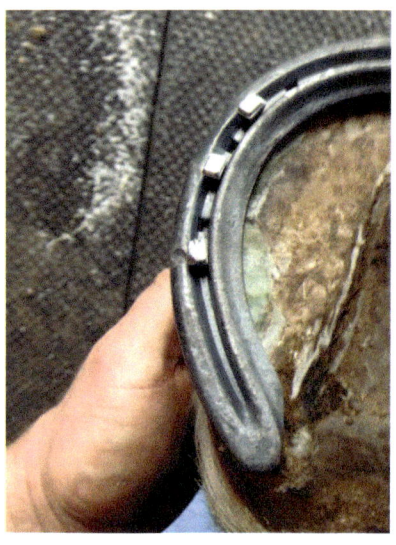

Fig. 13.13 The putty is held in position with a nailed on shoe that protects the cavity from further invasion.

Nail prick

A nail prick occurs when a horseshoe nail penetrates the sensitive structures of the hoof (Fig. 13.14). Usually, the horse will feel pain and snatch their foot away, when the nail is withdrawn there may be a smear of blood on the nail or blood may ooze from the nail hole.

Conditions of the white line

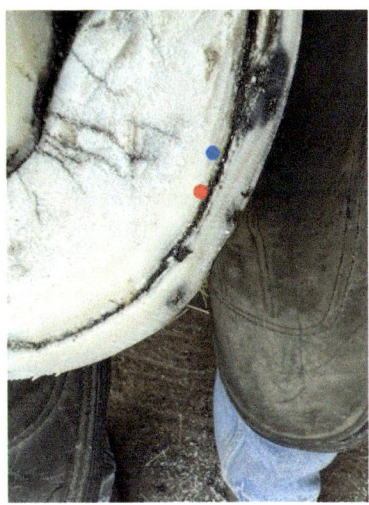

Fig. 13.14 The entry location of a nail prick (blue) and nail bind (red) to the solear aspect of the hoof.

Causes

Nail pricks are most likely to occur when:

- Working conditions are poor (bad light or rain).
- Thin, broken or excessively rasped hoof walls.
- Shoes fitted incorrectly.
- Coarse nail holes of the shoes fitted.

Treatment

Lameness will usually disappear when the nail is removed and in many cases, there are no complications. However, sometimes an inflammation develops due to tissue damage with lameness present along with an increased digital pulse and heat in the hoof. This will usually clear up in a few days if the hoof is poulticed and hot salt water bathed.

If an infection occurs the lameness will be severe and won't improve until drainage of the pus through the nail hole that penetrated the sensitive structures. Recovery is aided by hot poulticing and saltwater bathing. The horse's tetanus vaccination record should be checked and if not up to date, an anti toxin will be administered by a veterinary surgeon.

Prognosis

This tends to be a short term issue if the correct management procedures are followed as above. Usually, a maximum of two weeks off ridden work is required.

Nail bind

Nail binds occur when a nail has been driven too close to the sensitive laminae, creating pressure against it and causing lameness as a result of inflammation of sensitive structures. There will be heat in the hoof and an increased digital pulse.

Diagnosis

Location of the offending nail can be performed by using hoof testers and then removing each nail individually and inspecting the penetration of each nail once the shoe is removed.

Conditions of the white line

Treatment

If an infection develops, the shoe should be removed and hot poulticed with saltwater bathing similar to a nail prick. Ensure the horse's tetanus protection is up to date and if not, the veterinary surgeon will be required to administer an anti toxin.

Prognosis

As with a nail prick, the issue is short term and as long as any infection is cleared up, recovery time is quite short, and the horse can begin full work.

References

Butler, D & Butler, J. (2004) '*The Principles of Horseshoeing (P3)*', Doug Butler Enterprises: Colorado, USA.

Cole, S.D., Stefanovski, D., Towl, S. and Boyle, A.G. (2019), 'Factors associated with prolonged treatment days, increased veterinary visits and complications in horses with subsolar abscesses', *Veterinary Record*, Vol. 184, pp 251-257.

DeBowes, R.M. & Yovich, J.V. (1989) 'Penetrating Wounds, Abscesses, Gravel, and Bruising of the Equine Foot', *Veterinary Clinics of North America: Equine Practice*, Vol. 5, No.1, pp 179-194.

Ireland, J.L, McGowan, C.M, Clegg, P.D., Chandler, K.J. & Pinchbeck, G.L. (2012) 'A survey of health care and disease in geriatric horses aged 30years or older', *The Veterinary Journal*, Vol. 192, No. 1, pp 57-64.

Kuwano, A., Yoshihara, T., Takatori, K. and Kosuge, J. (1998), 'Onychomycosis in white line disease in horses: pathology, mycology and clinical features' *Equine Veterinary Journal*, Vol. 30, pp 27-35.

Moyer, W. (2003) 'Hoof wall defects: chronic hoof wall separations and hoof wall cracks' *Veterinary Clinics: Equine Practice*, Vol. *19*, No. 2, pp 463-477.

Trayhorn, D. (2019) 'To poultice or not to poultice?' *Equine Health*, Vol.49, pp 22-24.

Glossary of terms

The list of terms described below is used to describe some terms found within this book, some may have been explained within the chapters and therefore be omitted from the list.

Orientation and location terms

Distal: Away from the centre of the body towards the bearing border.

Dorsal: The front of the hoof.

Dorsopalmaro: Radiograph view looking from the front of the hoof.

Lateral: Away from the midline of the horse.

Medial: Towards the midline of the horse.

Mediolateral: Side to side comparison of the medial and lateral aspects of the hoof.

Palmar: The rear of the front hoof.

Plantar: The rear of the hind hoof.

Proximal: Towards the body, away from the hoof.

Solear: The underside of the hoof including the sole and frog.

Abbreviations

AFD: Acquired Flexoral Deformity.

DDFT: Deep Digital Flexor Tendon.

EMS: Equine Metabolic Syndrome.

PPID: Pituitary Pars Intermedia Disfunction.

General Terms

Abscess: A localised infection of the sensitive tissues of the hoof.

Acquired Flexoral Deformity (AFD): A deviation of the limb in the sagittal plane that leads to a club foot.

Antifungal: Inhibit microbiotic growth.

Arthritis: Inflammation or swelling of one or more joints.

Bilateral: Both sides of a hoof or a pair of limbs.

Breakover: The beginning of the stride when the toe is still on the ground whilst the heels are lifted.

Glossary of terms

Bruise: The rupturing of blood vessels within sensitive structures of the hoof as a result of trauma.

Bursa: A sac that releases synovial fluid to keep a joint lubricated.

Canker: A rare hypertrophy of the frog caused by a severe infection.

Caulkin: A turned down section of a horseshoe to provide extra grip.

Central Sulcis: The portion of the middle of the frog from its most rear extremity to the centre of the solear aspect.

Clubfoot: An upright hoof with a broken forward hoof pastern axis.

Coffin bone: The most distal bone in each limb that is found within the hoof capsule and resembles the shape of the hoof.

Coffin joint: The most distal joint in the limb made up of the coffin bone, navicular bone and short pastern bone.

Collapsed heels: A hoof with a low hoof wall angle and lack of any heel development along with a broken back hoof pastern axis.

Collateral: Either side or side by side

Conformation: The shape of a body part or parts.

Contralateral limb: The limb opposite the one that suffered the original patholody

Corium: A collection of blood vessels, lymphatic vessels and nerve endings that grow horn.

Crossfiring: A gait abnormality where diagonal feet collide.

Exercise: Controlled physical exertion.

Extension: A shoe that continues beyond the distal border of the hoof wall to impose symmetry on an asymmetrical hoof.

Foal: A young horse of either sex.

Foot: The entire hoof capsule and the structures contained within it.

Grass crack: A split in the hoof wall originating at the distal wall and travelling towards the top of the hoof.

Grip: Resistance to slide during the impact and stance phase of the stride

Impact phase: The first point of contact the hoof makes with the ground.

Hoof: The covering of the digit made up of a horny structure.

Hoof balance: A term used to describe the shape of the hoof in relation to the limb and dynamic locomotion.

Hoof pastern axis: The alignment of the pastern with the hoof wall angle that can be straight, broken backwards or broken forwards.

Glossary of terms

Laminae: The structures that suspends the horse's bodyweight within the hoof capsule effectively binding the coffin bone to the hoof wall.

Laminitis: An inflammation of the dermal laminae of the hoof.

Limb: The projecting paired appendages of the body that are used for locomotion.

Navicular bone: A small bone found behind the coffin bone that provides a fulcrum point for the deep digital flexor tendon to pass over.

Ossification: The change of soft tissues such as cartilage into bone.

Pathology: Alterations to the hoof caused by disease or trauma.

Pastern: The region between the fetlock and hoof.

Radiograph: An image that is produced by artificially generated radiation that passes through opaque matter so only dense objects such as bone can be visible on the image.

Sandcrack: A split originating from the coronary band and travelling towards the bottom of the hoof wall.

Sheared heel: Where there is a split from the central sulcis of the frog that extends into the skin and the heels move independently.

Sidebone: An ossification of the collateral cartilages of the hoof

Stay apparatus: The configuration of anatomical structures that allow the horse to rest whilst standing.

Tendon: Strong fibrous tissue that connects muscle to bone.

Toxaemia: A toxic reaction in the body to a foreign mass in the blood and lymphatic system.

Transphyseal bridging: The process of applying screws to one side of a joint to slow down development.

Trimming: The removal of excess horn using hoof knives, nippers and rasps

Unilateral: One side of a

Varus: A medial deviation of the limb from either the knee or fetlock.

Valgus: A lateral deviation of the limb from either the knee or fetlock.

Vertical axis rotation: An inward or outward rotation of an entire limb.

White line: The junction between the sole and hoof wall.

Index

Abscess 203-207

Amino acids 59

Angular limb deformities 70-73, 80-81

Arena surfaces 39-43

Arteries 14-16

Barefoot 35-36, 135, 136, 137

Bars 6

Bones 9-11

Breakover 103-104, 123-124, 125

Broken back hoof pastern axis 75-79, 90-91, 113-116

Broken forward hoof pastern axis 75-79, 90-91, 113-116

Brushing 125-126

Calcium 54

Camped under 81-82

Canker 174-177

Carpal/fetlock varus 72, 81

Carpal/fetlock valgus 71-72, 80

Coria 13 – 14

Coronary band 6, 13, 185

Coronitis 195

Cow hocked 82-83

Cartilage 12

Club foot 116-118

Cocksfoot 47

Coffin joint arthritis 152

Collateral ligament injury 134-135

Composite shoes 37-39

Contracted tendons 68-70

Copper 57

Coria 13-14

Corn 165-166

Coronary band 6

Crossfire 127

CT scan 100

Cushings disease 141

Cushions of the hoof 13

Dorso Palmar balance 90-91

Deep digital flexor tendon injury 135-136

Equine metabolic syndrome 144-145

False quarter 193

Fescues 47

Flexural flaccidity 67-68

Foal deformities 66-73

Forging 125

Frog 5, 171-172

Frog, atrophy 181-182

Frog, exfoliating 180

Index

Frog, granuloma 178-179

Frog, maggots 179

Frog, stave 179-180

Gait analysis 100-107

Grass 52-53

Grass crack 186-187

Gravel tracks 210-212

Growth plate 65-67

Growth ring 195-196

Hay 47-51

Hay analysis 48-51

Haylage 48

Heel 6

Heel bulbs 6

Hindgut 60-62

Hoof avulsion 190-192

Hoof boots 36 - 37

Hoof dressing 31 – 32

Hoof sloughing 147

Hoof wall 6, 185-186

Hoof wall bruise 196-197

Hoof wall, concussive trauma 199-200

Hoof wall cracks 186

Hoof wall separation syndrome 198-199

Horizontal crack 190

Iodine 58

Iron 58

Joints 10, 11

Keratoma 193-195

Keratin 59-60

Lameness 19 – 20

Laminitis 141 – 151

Laminitis, endocrinopathic 144-146

Laminitis, supporting limb 146

Laminitis, toxaemia 146

Laminitis, trauma induced 146

Landing phase 102-103

Ligament 18-19, 133

Lysine 59

Macrominerals 54-56

Magnesium 56

Manganese 58

Meadow hay 48

Medio-lateral balance 87-89, 111-113

Methylsulphanylmethane 56

Methionine 59

Microminerals 56-58

Midstance 103

Minerals 53-54

MRI 99

Index

Nail bind 213

Nail prick 212-213

Navicular syndrome 155-159

Neglected feet 26 - 27

Nerves 17 - 18

Nerve block 98

Overreach 29-31, 124-125

Pedal bone fracture 153-154

Pedal osteitis 159-160

Periople 6, 200

Phosphorus 54

Posture 119-120

Potassium 54

Poultice 205-207

Protein 59-60

Quarter 6

Quarter crack 189-190

Radiograph 94-98, 112, 147

Retracted sole 164-165

Ryegrass 48

Removing a shoe 24 - 26

Sandcrack 187-188

Seedy toe 209-210

Selenium 57-58

Shoe wear 92

Sidebone 154-155

Sodium 55

Soft tissue injury 137

Soil 53

Sole 6, 163

Sole bruise 165

Sole puncture 28 - 29, 166-167

Sole, under run 167

Solar crena marginilis 197-198

Sheared heels 177-178

Slipping 127-129

Stride timings 104

Studs 128-130

Sulphur 55

Swing phase 101-102

Tendon 11, 133

Thrush 172-173

Timothy hay 47

Tripping 123-124

Toe 6

Toe drag 126

Track systems 34 - 35

Tread 192-193

Type 1 founder 147-148

Type 2 founder 148

Index

Veins 14, 16–17

Venogram 99-100

Vermin damage 197

Vertical axis rotation 74

Vitamin 60

Vitamin A 60

Vitamin B 60

Vitamin E 60

Water 51-52

Wedges 115-116

White line 5, 203

White line disease 207-209

Windswept foal 72-73

Zinc 56